Tips and Tricks in Endocrine Surg

DATE DUE

John C. Watkinson • David M. Scott-Coombes
Editors

Neil Sharma • Michael J. Stechman
Shahzada K. Ahmed
Associate Editors

Tips and Tricks
in Endocrine Surgery

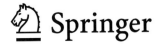 Springer

Editors
John C. Watkinson
ENT Department
Queen Elizabeth Hospital
Birmingham, UK

David M. Scott-Coombes, MS, FRCS
Department of Endocrine Surgery
University Hospital of Wales
Cardiff, UK

Associate Editors
Neil Sharma, MBChB, MRCS, DOHNS
Department of Otolaryngology
Head and Neck Surgery
University Hospital North Staffordshire
Newcastle-under-Lyme, UK

Shahzada K. Ahmed
Department of Ear, Nose and Throat Surgery
Queen Elizabeth Hospital Birmingham
University Hospital Birmingham NHS
Foundation Trust
Birmingham, UK

Michael J. Stechman, MBChB, MD
Department of Endocrine Surgery
University Hospital of Wales
Cardiff, UK

ISBN 978-0-85729-982-6   ISBN 978-1-4471-2146-6   (eBook)
DOI 10.1007/978-1-4471-2146-6
Springer London Heidelberg New York Dordrecht

Library of Congress Control Number: 2013950912

Foreword

In spite of a somewhat protracted and tortuous development, endocrine surgery has now come of age with its recognition and acceptance as a true surgical speciality in its own right.

It is difficult to determine at which point exactly this event occurred, but it was probably sometime in the 1960s and 1970s when surgeons began to regard the endocrine system as a whole, appreciated the need to work closely with other disciplines (endocrinologists, biochemists, radiologists, pathologists, nuclear medicine specialists, basic scientists, etc.), and also began to publish books and journals devoted to the subject. Postgraduate courses in endocrine surgery started to appear and very soon national and international associations were born.

Dramatic progress in the basic science underlying the speciality, particularly in the areas of biochemistry, molecular biology, and genetics, has placed unique demands upon the endocrine surgeon and emphasized the imperative to continually keep abreast of the latest information and knowledge. A veritable explosion of endoscopic and minimally invasive surgical advances has placed additional pressures upon the endocrine surgeon to keep up-to-date and remain at the forefront of his speciality.

The standard textbook has always fulfilled an important function in the communication of new knowledge, but with the arrival of the digital age and the ever-expanding role of the Internet and rapid electronic information transfer, some might consider the place of the traditional textbook to be under threat.

However, I believe that there is still an important role for the concise focused text which can provide the reader with instant, easily accessible advice and guidance.

This book, *Tips and Tricks in Endocrine Surgery*, is such a text and will certainly fill a vacant niche in the literature. Its publication will add to the legitimacy of the debate regarding the ideal educational medium. It is always difficult to decide upon the precise type of audience to which such a text should be directed. This book will be of particular value to the higher surgical trainee in endocrine surgery as well as the established consultant.

The contributors have been handpicked across the breadth of the speciality, including otorhinolaryngologists with expertise in thyroid and parathyroid surgery.

Indeed the professional credentials of the two extremely experienced coeditors testify to this cross-speciality cooperation. There is an excellent balance of contributions from surgeons and medical endocrinologists, including a rare finding in such a book of chapters addressing disorders of the pituitary.

It might be thought invidious to single out any particular chapter for comment, but there are several scholarly highlights, particularly in the sections describing surgical techniques for open and minimally invasive adrenalectomy, which are worthy of mention. These chapters provide exceptional detail and are full of tips, tricks, and pearls of wisdom completely in keeping with both the title and ethos of the book.

In a multiauthor book it is challenging to establish a uniform style and format throughout. However, in *Tips and Tricks in Endocrine Surgery*, the contributors and editors have succeeded in producing an academically credible text which is extremely readable, comprehensive and detailed, and full of sound practical advice which will undoubtedly have the potential to contribute to the provision of better and safer clinical care.

Throughout the book there are many references to the importance of team work and a multidisciplinary approach to difficult and complex endocrine problems. It is worth remembering that this is not a new concept in surgery. The famous Dr. Charles H. Mayo, a veritable doyen of thyroid surgery at the Mayo Clinic, wisely said, "The keynote of progress in the twentieth century is system and organization – in other words, 'team work.'" Few would today disagree with this sentiment.

I hope that Scott-Coombes and Watkinson's book will join the standard texts in the quest for provision of a continuum of information and opinion in the speciality. I enthusiastically recommend it to all endocrine surgeons.

Wales, UK   Malcolm H. Wheeler, MD, FRCS

Preface

This book was conceived from discussions between us about surgical teaching and multidisciplinary working. We believe there is still a place in the modern era for a text that simplifies a subject with a series of learning points, generated from the expert contribution of a number of specialities. This book aims to do just that. An international multidisciplinary faculty has combined to bring together the relevant endocrine topics, and the algebraic generic sum of their wisdom, learning, and experience means that anyone reading this text can do so in the confidence of knowing that the subject essentials will be both up-to-date and comprehensive.

Have a good read and spread the word!

Birmingham, UK   John C. Watkinson
Cardiff, UK   David M. Scott-Coombes, MS, FRCS

Contents

Contributors

Shahzada K. Ahmed Department of Ear, Nose and Throat Surgery, Queen Elizabeth Hospital Birmingham, University Hospital Birmingham NHS Foundation Trust, Birmingham, UK

M.A. Alzahrani Otolaryngology – Head and Neck Surgery, Massachusetts Eye and Ear Infirmary, Boston, MA, USA

Wiebke Arlt, MD, DSc, FRCP, FMedSci Department of Endocrinology, Centre for Endocrinology, Diabetes and Metabolism (CEDAM), School of Clinical and Experimental Medicine, University of Birmingham, Birmingham, West Midlands, UK

Stephen L. Atkin, MBBS, FRCP, PhD Department of Diabetes, Endocrinology and Metabolism, University of Hull, Hull Royal Infirmary, Hull, UK

Mo Aye, MBBS, FRCP, FRCPEdin Department of Diabetes, Endocrinology and Metabolism, Centre for Metabolic Bone Disease Hull and East Yorkshire Hospitals NHS Trust, Hull Royal Infirmary, Hull, UK

John Ayuk, MD, MRCP Department of Endocrinology, Queen Elizabeth Hospital Birmingham, Birmingham, West Midlands, UK

University of Birmingham and Queen Elizabeth Hospital Birmingham, University Hospital Birmingham NHS Foundation Trust, Birmingham, UK

Thomas J. Beech, MBChB, MSc, DOHNS, FRCS ENT Department, University Hospital Birmingham, Birmingham, West Midlands, UK

Tara D. Barwick, MSc, MRCP, FRCR Department of Imaging, Imperial College Healthcare NHS Trust, Hammersmith Hospital, London, UK

Kristien Boelaert, MD, PhD, MRCP Department of Endocrinology, University Hospital Birmingham, Birmingham, UK

Centre for Endocrinology, Diabetes and Metabolism, Institute of Biomedical Research, School of Clinical and Experimental Medicine, University of Birmingham, Birmingham, UK

Bruno Carnaille, MD Department of Endocrine Surgery, University Hospital, Hopital Huriez, Lille, France

Swarupsinh V. Chavda Department of Neuroradiology, Queen Elizabeth Hospital Birmingham, University Hospital Birmingham NHS Foundation Trust, Birmingham, UK

Ioannis Christakis Department of Thyroid and Endocrine Surgery, Imperial College NHS Trust, Hammersmith Campus, London, UK

Penelope M. Clark, MSc, PhD, FRCPath Regional Endocrine Laboratory, Clinical Laboratory Services, Queen Elizabeth Hospital Birmingham, Birmingham, West Midlands, UK

University of Birmingham and Queen Elizabeth Hospital Birmingham, University Hospital Birmingham NHS Foundation Trust, Birmingham, UK

Thomas Clerici, MD Deparament of Surgery, Kantonsspital St. Gallen, St. Gallen, Switzerland

Helen Cocks, MD, MBChB, FRCS Department of Otolaryngology, City Hospitals Sunderland NHS Trust, Sunderland, UK

Caroline Connolly, MBChB, FRCR Department of Oncology, Queen Elizabeth Hospital Cancer Centre, Birmingham, West Midlands, UK

Vasilis A. Constantinides Department of Thyroid and Endocrine Surgery, Imperial College NHS Trust, Hammersmith Campus, London, UK

Jeremy Davis, MBBS, FRCS ENT Department, Medway Maritime Hospital, Gillingham, Kent, UK

R. James England, MBChB, FRCS (ORL-HNS) Department of ENT/Head and Neck Surgery, Hull and East Yorkshire Hospitals NHS Trust, Castle Hill Hospital, Cottingham, East Riding of Yorkshire, UK

Jeremy Freeman Department of Otolaryngology, Head and Neck Surgery, Mount Sinai Hospital, Toronto, Canada

Ajith Paulose George, MBChB, FRCS (ORL-HNS) Department of Otolaryngology, Head and Neck Surgery, Russells Hall Hospital, Dudley, West Midlands, Birmingham Heartlands Hospital, UK

John Glaholm Department of Oncology, Queen Elizabeth Hospital Cancer Centre, Birmingham, West Midlands, UK

Osama Al Hamarneh, MBBS, MRCS, DOHNS, MD ENT Department, Queen Elizabeth Hospital, Birmingham, West Midlands, UK

Meredydd Harries Department of Otolaryngology, Head and Neck Surgery, Royal Sussex County Hospital, Brighton, UK

Barney Harrison, MBBS, MS, FRCS Eng Department of Endocrine Surgery, Royal Hallamshire Hospital, Sheffield, UK

Ian D. Hay Division of Endocrinology, Diabetes, Metabolism, and Nutrition, Mayo Clinic, Rochester, MN, USA

Per Hellman, MD, PhD Department of Surgical Sciences, Uppsala University, Uppsala, Sweden

James E. Jackson, FRCP, FRCR Department of Imaging, Hammersmith Hospital, London, UK

Sharan Jayaram Department of Otolaryngology, Head and Neck Surgery, University Hospital Birmingham, Birmingham, UK

Alan Johnson Department of Ear, Nose and Throat Surgery, Queen Elizabeth Hospital Birmingham, University Hospital Birmingham NHS Foundation Trust, Birmingham, UK

Maninder Singh Kalkat, FRCS Department of Thoracic Surgery, Birmingham Heartlands Hospital, UK

Dae Kim Department of Otolaryngology, Head and Neck Surgery, Queen Alexandra Hospital, Portsmouth, UK

Judit Konya, MBBS Department of Diabetes, Endocrinology and Metabolism, University of Hull, Hull Royal Infirmary, Hull, UK

Sonia Kumar, MRCS (Eng), DOHNS Department of Otolaryngology, Royal Berkshire Hospital, Reading, Berkshire, UK

Andrew Lansdown Department of Endocrine Sciences, Institute of Molecular and Experimental Medicine, Centre for Endocrine and Diabetes Sciences, School of Medicine, Cardiff University, Cardiff, UK

Thomas W. J. Lennard, MBBS, FRCS, MD Department of Surgery, Royal Victoria Infirmary, Newcastle Upon Tyne, UK

Lisha McClelland Department of Otolaryngology, Queen Elizabeth Hospital Birmingham, University Hospital Birmingham NHS Foundation Trust, Birmingham, UK

Karim Meeran Department of Endocrinology, Imperial Centre for Endocrinology, Hammersmith Hospital Campus, London, UK

Hisham Mehanna, PhD, BMedSc (hons), MBChB (hons), FRCS, FRCS (ORL-HNS) Department of Head and Neck Surgery, School of Cancer Sciences, Institute of Head and Neck Studies and Education, University of Birmingham, Birmingham, UK

Radu Mihai, MD, PhD, FRCS Department of Endocrine Surgery, John Radcliffe Hospital, Oxford, UK

Rosalind Mitchell Department of Neurosurgery, Queen Elizabeth Hospital Birmingham, University Hospital Birmingham NHS Foundation Trust, Birmingham, UK

Ram Moorthy, FRCS (ORL-HNS) Otolaryngology- Head and Neck Surgery, ENT, Heatherwood and Wexham Park Hospitals NHS Trust, Wexham Park Hospital, Wexham Berkshire, UK

Fausto Palazzo Department of Thyroid and Endocrine Surgery, Imperial College NHS Trust, Hammersmith Campus, London, UK

Gregory W. Randolph, MD Otolaryngology – Head and Neck Surgery, Massachusetts Eye and Ear Infirmary, Boston, MA, USA

Aled Rees, FRCP, PhD Department of Endocrine Sciences, Institute of Molecular and Experimental Medicine, Centre for Endocrine and Diabetes Sciences, School of Medicine, Cardiff University, Cardiff, UK

Scott Russell Department of Anaethestics, Queen Elizabeth Hospital, Birmingham, UK

Gregory P. Sadler, MD, FRCS Gen Surg (Eng) Department of Endocrine Surgery, John Radcliffe Hospital, Oxford, UK

Bruno Schmied, MD Deparament of Surgery, Kantonsspital St. Gallen, St. Gallen, Switzerland

David M. Scott-Coombes, MS, FRCS Department of Endocrine Surgery, University Hospital of Wales, Cardiff, UK

Ashok Shaha Jatin P. Shah Chair in Head and Neck Surgery and Oncology, Memorial Sloan-Kettering Cancer Center, New York, USA

Neil Sharma, MBChB, MRCS, DOHNS Department of Otolaryngology, Head and Neck Surgery, University Hospital North Staffordshire, Newcastle-under-Lyme, UK

Joel Anthony Smith, FRCS (ORL-HNS), MBChB, BMedSc, DOHNS Department of Otolaryngology, Head and Neck Surgery, University Hospital Birmingham, Queen Elizabeth Medical Centre, Birmingham, West Midlands, UK

Peter Stålberg, MD, PhD Department of Surgical Sciences, Uppsala University, Uppsala, Sweden

Michael J. Stechman, MBChB, MD Department of Endocrine Surgery, University Hospital of Wales, Cardiff, UK

Neil Tolley, MD, FRCS Department of Otolaryngology, Head and Neck Surgery, Imperial College Healthcare NHS Trust, St Mary's Hospital, London, UK

Rachel Troke Department of Endocrinology, Imperial Centre for Endocrinology, Hammersmith Hospital Campus, London, UK

John C. Watkinson ENT Department, Queen Elizabeth Hospital, Birmingham, UK

Richard Wight Department of Otolaryngology, Head and Neck Surgery, James Cook University Hospital, Middlesbrough, UK

Beng K. Yap, MBChB, FRCP, FRCR Department of Clinical Oncology, The Christie NHS Foundation Trust, Manchester, Lancashire, UK

Part I
Adrenal

Chapter 1
Adrenal and Paraganglioma: Presentation, Assessment, and Diagnosis

Andrew Lansdown and Aled Rees

- The adrenal cortex represents 90 % of the gland and is divided into three zones:
  - Zona glomerulosa (outer), aldosterone-secreting
  - Zona fasciculata (intermediate), cortisol-secreting
  - Zona reticularis (inner), androgen-secreting
- The medulla is the inner core of the gland and secretes around 20 % noradrenaline and 80 % adrenaline.

Cushing's Syndrome

Presentation

- Typically affects women (4:1) at a young age (30–40 years).
- A high index of suspicion is required for early diagnosis and treatment.
- Left untreated, Cushing's syndrome is associated with a high mortality (up to 50 % within 5 years), principally from cardio-/cerebrovascular disease.
- Clinical features include:

  - Central weight gain, buffalo hump, plethoric "moon" face 70–80 %
  - Hypertension 70–80 %
  - Skin thinning, purple striae, easy bruising, facial plethora 60–70 %
  - Psychological symptoms, depression, irritability 60–70 %

A. Lansdown • A. Rees, FRCP, PhD (✉)
Department of Endocrine Sciences, Institute of Molecular
and Experimental Medicine, Centre for Endocrine
and Diabetes Sciences, School of Medicine,
Cardiff University, Cardiff CF14 4XN, UK
e-mail: reesda@cf.ac.uk

J.C. Watkinson, D.M. Scott-Coombes (eds.), *Tips and Tricks in Endocrine Surgery*,
DOI 10.1007/978-1-4471-2146-6_1, © Springer-Verlag London 2014

- Proximal myopathy 50–60 %
- Oligomenorrhea/impotence 50–60 %
- Hirsutism and acne 40–70 %

- Consider the diagnosis particularly if osteoporosis and/or hypertension is present in a young person.
- "Subclinical" Cushing's syndrome refers to the presence of mild, autonomous hypercortisolism without specific clinical signs of cortisol excess; this typically occurs in the context of incidentally discovered adrenal adenomas (adrenal "incidentalomas").
- Subclinical Cushing's syndrome may be associated with an increased prevalence of hypertension and impaired glucose tolerance, but the natural history and optimal management is presently unclear.
- Cushing's syndrome from ectopic ACTH secretion is usually due to malignancy and presents with weight loss, metabolic disturbances (hypokalemic alkalosis), and severe myopathy.

Assessment

- Features which best discriminate Cushing's syndrome from simple, generalized obesity include proximal myopathy and thinning of the skin/easy bruising.
- Full assessment of metabolic and cardiovascular status should be undertaken.
- Blood pressure should be measured and controlled appropriately.
- Patients should be screened and treated for diabetes mellitus and any underlying infection.

Diagnosis

1. Is hypercortisolism present?

   Screening tests:

   - Overnight dexamethasone suppression test. Give 1 mg oral dexamethasone at 11 p.m. and measure serum cortisol at 9 a.m. the following morning. Normal response is complete cortisol suppression (<50 nmol/l). High sensitivity (95 %) and moderate specificity (85 %); false positive with oral contraceptive, hormone replacement therapy and liver enzyme inducers.
   - Late night salivary cortisol. Convenient, measured at 11 p.m. or midnight. High sensitivity but low specificity.
   - Urinary free cortisol – at least two collections needed to avoid missing mild disease. False negative with renal failure. Low specificity: false positive in alcoholism, depression, and polycystic ovary syndrome.
   - A combination of tests is usually required to make the diagnosis.

Confirmatory tests:

- Low-dose dexamethasone suppression. Administer 0.5 mg dexamethasone 6 hourly for 48 h. Normal response is complete cortisol suppression (<50 nmol/l). High sensitivity and specificity (98 %) when interpreted at this cortisol cutoff.

2. What is the cause of hypercortisolism?

Tests to confirm source:

- Tests to confirm the source should only be undertaken when a diagnosis of hypercortisolism is established.
- First step is to measure plasma ACTH. Levels <5 pg/ml on several occasions indicate ACTH-independent disease; levels >15 pg/ml indicate likely ACTH-dependent source.
- In cases where ACTH independence is confirmed, CT is indicated to establish an adrenal lesion.
- In ACTH-dependent Cushing's syndrome, MRI pituitary may demonstrate a pituitary adenoma.
- Bilateral inferior petrosal sinus sampling (BIPSS) can be used to differentiate between a pituitary and ectopic ACTH source. High sensitivity and specificity (95 %).
- Chest X-ray may localize an ectopic source (mandatory in all smokers).
- CT/MRI chest and abdomen is recommended to search for tumors associated with ectopic ACTH production when pituitary source excluded.

Medical Management

- In severe Cushing's syndrome, or where complications such as refractory hypertension or poorly controlled diabetes are present, medical treatment should be considered prior to surgery.
- Metyrapone (11-β-hydroxylase inhibitor), ketoconazole (imidazole antifungal), or etomidate alone or in combination can be used in these situations. Etomidate infusion requires ventilation on ICU.
- Liaison with endocrinologist is essential.

Conn's Syndrome

Presentation

- Moderate to severe hypertension, often refractory to treatment (three or more drugs) (systolic blood pressure 140–160 or diastolic blood pressure 90–99 mmHg) in a relatively young patient.

Table 1.1 Medications that may interfere with PAC: PRA ratio	Amiloride
	Estrogen (combined oral contraceptive pill, hormone replacement therapy)
	Diuretics
	ACE inhibitors
	Angiotensin II receptor blockers
	Dihydropyridine calcium channel blockers
	Heparin
	Lithium
	Nonsteroidal anti-inflammatory drugs (NSAIDs)

- Hypokalemia (serum K^+ <3.5 mmol/l) (50 %), with symptoms including fatigue, muscle cramps, thirst, polyuria, and nocturia, although commonly asymptomatic.
- 50 % are normokalemic.
- Increased risk of cardio-/cerebrovascular disease compared to essential hypertension.

Assessment

- Check blood pressure.
- U+E (hypokalemia, sodium upper end of normal or mildly elevated) with alkalosis.
- Indications for screening include adrenal incidentaloma with hypertension, refractory hypertension (on three or more drugs), severe hypertension (≥160 mmHg systolic and/or ≥100 mmHg diastolic), hypertension in a young adult (less than 40 years or strong family history), and hypokalemic alkalosis.

Diagnosis

- Liaise with endocrinologists.

  Screening tests:

  - Correct hypokalemia before collecting blood for aldosterone and renin.
  - Measure plasma aldosterone to plasma renin ratio (ARR).
  - Discontinue beta-blockers (2 weeks) and spironolactone (6 weeks) beforehand.
  - Other drugs may also affect interpretation but alpha-blockers do not (Table 1.1).
  - Plasma renin activity will typically be suppressed (<0.5 pmol/ml/h; normal 0.5–3.5) with a raised plasma aldosterone concentration >250 pmol/l. An ARR of >2,000 makes a diagnosis of Conn's syndrome very likely.

  Confirmatory tests:

  - These include the fludrocortisone suppression test and saline suppression test depending on local policy. Aldosterone fails to suppress in patients with primary hyperaldosteronism.

- High-resolution CT of the adrenal glands is required in patients with biochemically confirmed primary hyperaldosteronism. This may show a unilateral hypodense adenoma, bilateral hyperplasia/nodularity, unilateral adrenal thickening, or normal appearances.
- Other than in young (<40 years) patients with a typical presentation and confirmed (>1 cm) adenoma, all patients require lateralization of aldosterone secretion prior to surgery, principally because incidentalomas are common (4–7 % of the population), and there is a risk of misattributing the aldosterone excess to the adrenal adenoma.
- Adrenal venous sampling for primary hyperaldosteronism:
    - Samples are collected from the left and right adrenal veins, inferior vena cava, and peripheral blood pre- and post-synacthen stimulation.
    - An aldosterone to cortisol ratio of one adrenal vein versus the other of >4:1 is indicative of unilateral secretion, whereas a ratio of <3:1 is indicative of bilateral secretion.
- ^{11}C-metomidate PET-CT scanning may be a sensitive and specific noninvasive alternative to adrenal venous sampling for lateralizing aldosterone secretion by Conn's adenomas, but is not widely available.
- Testing for rare genetic causes (e.g., familial hyperaldosteronism type I or type II) may be necessary in certain circumstances (very early onset or family history of stroke or hypertension at a young age).

Medical Management

- Aldosterone receptor antagonists, such as spironolactone and eplerenone, can be used.
- Spironolactone can cause gynecomastia and reduced libido in men and menstrual disturbance in women.
- Eplerenone has a lower affinity for sex hormone receptors, hence is a useful alternative to spironolactone for men who develop gynecomastia, but has marginally inferior antihypertensive effects.
- Patients with Conn's syndrome may have coexisting essential hypertension and often need other antihypertensive treatment even after successful surgery.

Pheochromocytoma/Paraganglioma

Presentation

- Patients may be symptomatic or asymptomatic.
- Typical symptoms include sweating (60–70 %), sustained or episodic hypertension (>90 %), and headache (90 %).

- Other symptoms include pallor or flushing, palpitations, anxiety, panic attacks, and postural hypotension (due to decreased plasma volume).
- The presentation depends on the predominant catecholamine secreted by the tumor together with the pattern of release. Noradrenaline-secreting tumors tend to cause sustained hypertension, whereas tumors secreting adrenaline and nor-adrenaline often cause episodic hypertension. Rarely, dopamine-secreting tumors can cause hypotension.
- About 10 % of tumors are discovered incidentally on abdominal imaging under-taken for other reasons.
- Clinical signs are usually absent.

Assessment

- Assessment of blood pressure and cardiovascular status (including evidence of arrhythmias or left ventricular failure).
- Check for evidence of hypercalcemia and glucose intolerance.
- Screening for pheochromocytomas should be considered in:
  - Patients of a young age with hypertension
  - Patients with unexplained heart failure
  - Patients with classic episodic symptoms
  - Those with adrenal incidentalomas
  - Patients with a family history of von Hippel-Lindau (VHL) syndrome, mul-tiple endocrine neoplasia (MEN) 2A or 2B, type 1 neurofibromatosis (NF1), or inherited paraganglioma syndrome (due to mutation in one of the succinate dehydrogenase (*SDH*) genes)

Diagnosis

- Biochemical confirmation of elevated catecholamines and/or their metabolites is required.
- Measurement of plasma or urinary metanephrines (99 and 97 % sensitive) and plasma or urinary catecholamines (86 and 84 % sensitive) have superseded uri-nary vanillylmandelic acid (72 % sensitive).
- More than one measurement may be required because of intermittent tumor secretion.
- False positive results can occur with sympathomimetics, phenoxybenzamine, tricyclic antidepressants, and other drugs (Table 1.2).
- The initial imaging test of choice is CT or MRI of the abdomen/adrenals.
- If a tumor is not localized, ^{123}I-metaiodobenzylguanidine (^{123}I-MIBG) scanning and/or whole body imaging with CT or MRI is indicated.
- Ultrasound scanning is useful for surveillance of the neck in patients with inher-ited paraganglioma syndromes (due to mutations in the *SDHC* and *SDHD* genes).
- In special circumstances positron emission tomography may be indicated (see Chap. 4).

Table 1.2 Drugs known to increase catecholamine and metanephrine concentrations

Levodopa
Adrenergic receptor agonists, e.g., decongestants such as phenylephrine and ephedrine
Tricyclic antidepressants
Amphetamines
Buspirone and most psychoactive drugs
Prochlorperazine
Reserpine
Withdrawal from clonidine
Ethanol
Paracetamol (may interfere with plasma metanephrine assays)

- Up to 30 % of patients with pheochromocytoma/paraganglioma have a genetic cause for their disease (see Chap. 4). This is more likely in young patients (<50 years) or those presenting with malignant, bilateral, or extra-adrenal disease. Such patients should be referred for genetic testing.

Adrenal Incidentaloma

Presentation

- Defined as an adrenal tumor not suspected prior to the imaging procedure that led to its discovery.
- Overall 4 % prevalence, increasing to 7 % over the age of 70 years.
- At the time of diagnosis, up to 20 % of all incidentalomas may be endocrinologically active.

Assessment

- Larger tumors are more likely to be malignant, especially >6 cm diameter.
- The likelihood of endocrine overactivity increases with increasing size of the mass, except for aldosterone-producing adenomas with hypertension (typically <1 cm).
- Assessment should include examination for symptoms and signs of hormone excess and extra-adrenal malignancy.
- Questions for consideration are:
  - Is this an adrenal or extra-adrenal mass?
  - Is the adrenal mass a metastasis of a primary tumor?
  - Is the mass hormonally active?
  - Is there evidence of adrenocortical carcinoma (ACC)? The incidence of ACC at presentation is very low as is development with follow-up.

Diagnosis

- Biochemical evaluation should include:
    - Overnight dexamethasone suppression test
    - Measurement of renal function and electrolytes
    - ARR if hypertensive
    - Plasma or urinary metanephrines/catecholamines
- Urine steroid metabolomics may offer a novel, highly sensitive, and specific biomarker for distinguishing benign from malignant adrenal tumors but is not yet widely available.
- Measurement of Hounsfield units (HU) in an unenhanced CT is helpful in distinguishing benign from malignant disease. A threshold value of 10 HU has sensitivity and specificity for characterizing a lesion as benign of 71 and 98 %, respectively. Incidentalomas with >10 HU attenuation on unenhanced CT require more detailed review.
- Patients with a nonfunctioning adrenal mass should undergo follow-up CT or MRI at 6 months.
- Endocrinologically active tumors, tumors >4 cm, tumors showing imaging characteristics of malignancy (e.g., vascular invasion, lack of well-demarcated margins), and tumors showing significant growth should be removed.
- Patients with mild glucocorticoid autonomy ("subclinical Cushing's") should be assessed for possible complications related to cortisol excess (e.g., hypertension, type 2 diabetes, osteoporosis), and a decision on the need for surgery should be made on a case-by-case basis, in the absence of a robust evidence base with which to inform management.

Adrenocortical Carcinoma (ACC) (See Chap. 5)

Presentation

- Bimodal age distribution – children under 5 and adults 30–40 years old.
- In children most tumors are functional and may present with symptoms and signs of virilization, Cushing's syndrome, and precocious puberty.
- In adults, the most common presentation is rapidly progressing Cushing's syndrome, with or without virilization.
- In women, androgen-secreting ACCs may cause hirsutism, virilization, male-pattern baldness, and deepening of the voice.
- In males, rare estrogen-secreting adrenal tumors are invariably malignant and present with gynecomastia/testicular atrophy.
- Nonfunctional ACCs may present with abdominal/flank pain from local invasion or rarely may be detected incidentally.
- Occasionally patients may present with weight loss and fever.

Assessment

- Assess for signs and symptoms of Cushing's syndrome, virilization in women, Conn's syndrome (rare), or feminization in men (rare).

Diagnosis

- Biochemical assessment for evidence of glucocorticoid (see section on Cushing's syndrome), mineralocorticoid (see section on Conn's syndrome), or sex steroid excess, as well as metanephrine/catecholamine measurement.
- Measure sex steroids and steroid precursors including dehydroepiandrosterone-sulfate (DHEAS), 17-hydroxyprogesterone, androstenedione, testosterone, and 17-beta estradiol (latter only in men and postmenopausal women).
- CT or MRI: ACCs are typically >6 cm in size, heterogeneous with necrosis and calcification, and show evidence of local invasion. However, appearances are often nonspecific and may not discriminate from pheochromocytoma or extra-adrenal malignancy.
- ^{18}F-FDG PET scanning may provide additional information to define malignant potential, but this is not specific.
- High-resolution CT of the chest should also be performed prior to surgery to assess for the presence of metastases.
- Biopsy is rarely required and should never be undertaken without prior exclusion of a pheochromocytoma. A biopsy is not indicated in patients with an isolated adrenal mass due to the risks of needle-track metastasis and the difficulty in distinguishing benign from malignant pathology. A diagnostic biopsy may be required if the presence of extensive metastases precludes surgery or if malignant disease elsewhere raises the possibility of a non-adrenal primary tumor.
- Pathological assessment should be performed by an experienced pathologist.

Pearls and Pitfalls
Pearls

- Liaise closely with endocrinologists when assessing and diagnosing adrenal disease
- Beware of false-positive test results when investigating adrenal disorders
- A combination of biochemical and radiological investigations is usually required to make an accurate diagnosis of an adrenal lesion
- Do not presume that an adrenal adenoma is the cause of primary hyperaldosteronism without undertaking lateralization studies
- Cushing's syndrome should be approached with two questions: Is hypercortisolism present? What is the cause of hypercortisolism?

- Never proceed to surgery or biopsy of an adrenal mass without prior exclusion of a pheochromocytoma
- PET scanning using new tracers and urinary steroid metabolomics are emerging as novel tools in assessing the nature of adrenal lesions

Pitfalls

- All patients with paraganglioma and young patients (<50 years) with pheochromocytoma should undergo genetic testing for mutations in relevant susceptibility genes
- Preoperative medical preparation is often required in advance of adrenal surgery and is mandatory in patients with paraganglioma or pheochromocytoma

Further Reading

Burton TJ, Mackenzie IS, Balan K, Koo B, Bird N, Soloviev DV, Azizan EA, Aigbirhio F, Gurnell M, Brown MJ. Evaluation of the sensitivity and specificity of (11)C-metomidate positron emission tomography (PET)-CT for lateralizing aldosterone secretion by Conn's adenomas. J Clin Endocrinol Metab. 2012;97(1):100–9.

Lacroix A. Approach to the patient with adrenocortical carcinoma. J Clin Endocrinol Metab. 2010;95:4812–22.

Mulatero P, Monticone S, Bertello C, Tizzani D, Iannaccone A, Crudo V, Veglio F. Evaluation of primary aldosteronism. Curr Opin Endocrinol Diabetes Obes. 2010;17(3):188–93.

Nieman LK. Approach to the patient with an adrenal incidentaloma. J Clin Endocrinol Metab. 2010;95(9):4106–13.

Nieman LK, Biller BMK, Findling JW, Newell-Price J, Savage MO, Stewart PM, Montori VM. The diagnosis of Cushing's syndrome: an Endocrine Society Clinical Practice Guideline. J Clin Endocrinol Metab. 2008;93(5):1526–40.

Zeiger MA, Thompson GB, Duh QY, Hamrahian AH, Angelos P, Elaraj D, Fishman E, Kharlip J, American Association of Clinical Endocrinologists, American Association of Endocrine Surgeons. The American Association of Clinical Endocrinologists and American Association of Endocrine Surgeons medical guidelines for the management of adrenal incidentalomas. Endocr Pract. 2009;15 Suppl 1:1–20.

Chapter 2
Cushing's Disease and Syndrome

Thomas W.J. Lennard

Definition

Cushing's is characterized by increased levels of circulating glucocorticoids. There are two types:

- ACTH dependent due to either pituitary or ectopic ACTH secretion
- ACTH independent due to an autonomous adrenal excess production of corticosteroids from the zona fasciculata

    - 50 % benign adenoma
    - 50 % adrenocortical carcinoma (ACC)

The majority of patients (80 %) have ACTH (pituitary driven) dependent Cushing's disease.

Epidemiology

- A rare entity with a prevalence of ten cases per million of the population per year
- Peak presentation at 20–40 years
- More common in women

    Clinical features of the disease include:

- Truncal obesity and limb muscle wasting ("lemon on sticks").
- Facial plethora.
- Hirsutism.

T.W.J. Lennard, MBBS, FRCS, MD
Department of Surgery, Royal Victoria Infirmary,
Queen Victoria Road, Newcastle Upon Tyne NE1 4PL, UK
e-mail: t.w.j.lennard@ncl.ac.uk

J.C. Watkinson, D.M. Scott-Coombes (eds.), *Tips and Tricks in Endocrine Surgery*,
DOI 10.1007/978-1-4471-2146-6_2, © Springer-Verlag London 2014

- Menstrual disorders.
- Myopathy.
- Striae.
- Acne.
- Psychological symptoms.
- Congestive heart failure.
- Hypertension.
- Secondary diabetes mellitus.
- ACC may present with local symptoms of compression by adrenal mass.
- Patients with ectopic acth driven disease are usually pigmented.

Pathology

- Benign adenoma.
- Malignant tumor – size, local invasion, but as with pheochromocytoma, definitive diagnosis can be difficult if there is no local invasion or metastasis.
- "Atypical" adenoma vs. carcinoma (former in children may behave less aggressively; latter in adults and has poor prognosis).
- Neuroendocrine tumor (NET) secreting ACTH.

Investigation and Diagnosis

Once clinical suspicion has been raised, the diagnosis is confirmed with biochemical investigations. Work closely with endocrinologists (see Chap. 1).

- 24-h urinary free cortisol excretion.
- The normal cortisol diurnal rhythm (morning and midnight) usually becomes lost.
- ACTH levels will determine whether this is pituitary driven or adrenal in origin.
- Low-dose dexamethasone suppression test exploits the loss of negative feedback by the adrenal to the pituitary.

Once the biochemical diagnosis is confirmed, localization of the source of the problem is required. For ACTH-dependent Cushing's disease, this will require an MRI or CT of the pituitary gland. Petrosal venous sampling may be required in patients for whom no tumor is identified. For adrenal-driven hypercortisolism, a CT or MRI of the adrenal glands is the imaging modality of choice (Fig. 2.1).

Medical Management

- Medical therapy may be required in severe fulminating Cushing's to permit surgery or as a bridge to surgical resection (see Chap. 1).

Fig. 2.1 Contrast-enhanced CT scan in a patient with Cushing's syndrome demonstrating a left primary adrenal tumor and a synchronous metastasis in the right lobe of the liver

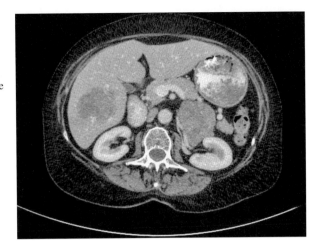

Indications for Surgery

Cushing's syndrome – surgery should be considered in all patients if fit.

Cushing's disease after failed pituitary surgery – bilateral adrenalectomy.

Subclinical Cushing's – more controversial but if evidence of metabolic syndrome (MS) and adrenal mass/bulky adrenals, surgery should be discussed as it may improve MS manifestations.

Surgery

Cushing's Disease

If the patient has got a pituitary tumor, then clearly surgery via a direct approach to that, usually transsphenoidal, will be required (see Chap. 5).

Cushing's Syndrome

Preoperative Considerations

- Is the tumor co-secreting additional hormones?

    - 24-h urinary or plasma metanephrines in patients with hypertension

- Could the tumor be malignant? Carcinomas of the adrenal gland commonly present with corticosteroid excess, often in combination with other hormones. It is important not to miss a carcinoma of the adrenal gland presenting as Cushing's syndrome, as the planned surgical approach may need to be adjusted if this is the likely diagnosis.

- Achieve optimal preoperative control of hypertension, diabetes, and improving muscle strength where possible.
- Patients are susceptible to infection with high doses of circulating steroids; wound healing will also be inhibited. It is often advisable, therefore, in these circumstances to block the effect of the steroids with drugs such as ketoconazole before surgery, aiming to allow the operation to take place in a patient who is not suffering from the gross metabolic consequences of hypercortisolism.
- Patients should receive thromboprophylaxis according to NICE guidelines.
- Patients with Cushing's are susceptible to peptic ulcers, and prophylaxis should be considered.

Operative Considerations

- Very careful (gentle) positioning of the patient who may have skin that easily bruises as well as severe osteoporosis. All pressure points must be carefully protected.
- Prophylactic antibiotics should be prescribed.
- Laparoscopic surgery (via either a transperitoneal or a posterior approach) for an adrenal adenoma is the ideal approach. Open surgery should be the approach if malignancy is suspected (see Chap. 5).
- Platelet function is suppressed in the presence of high steroid levels. Be aware that the liver bruises easily and subcapsular hematomas can readily develop during dissection.
- Crucial to avoid capsular breach or incomplete excision in Cushing's disease with failed pituitary surgery or NET-related Cushing's due to risk of hypertrophy of remnants and recurrent disease.

Complications and Outcomes

Postoperative Considerations

- Steroid replacement. The remaining adrenal gland, if it is in situ, will be suppressed, and the patient will require steroid support until the pituitary adrenal access has restored itself to normal as determined by short synacthen test(s).
- Supraphysiological levels of steroids can both cause complications and mask the manifestations of sepsis. The surgeon should have a heightened awareness for the possibility of complications (Table 2.1).
- The postoperative hospital length of stay is longer for this group of patients compared with other indications for adrenalectomy. Nevertheless the laparoscopic approach has had a huge benefit for these patients.
- An improvement in the physical signs from Cushing's disease or syndrome after surgery may take up to 2 years to complete.

Table 2.1 Complications of surgery for Cushing's

Immediate	Early	Late
Bleeding – IVC or left renal vein. May require conversion to open surgery	Adrenal bed hematoma Wound hematoma Wound infection	Port site or incisional hernia
Hemodynamic instability – hypertensive stroke or MI, arrhythmia, cardiac arrest	Ileus Respiratory or urinary tract infection Thromboembolic event	Local or distant recurrence due to undiagnosed malignant disease
Thermal injury to adjacent bowel, blood vessels, or organs, e.g., spleen.	Addisonian crisis Peptic ulcer disease	Addisonian crisis in steroid dependent patients
	Continued bleeding – rare	

Patients with malignant disease are referred for adjuvant chemotherapy but have a poor prognosis.

Pearls and Pitfalls
Pearls

- Complete biochemical analysis is essential to ensure there is no co-secretion of other hormones with glucocorticoids.
- Be careful not to miss an adrenal cortical cancer.
- Good quality imaging of the pituitary and the adrenal glands is required.
- Do not fail to optimize DVT prevention.
- Work closely with endocrinologists for diagnosis and perioperative management.
- Do not forget to give postoperative steroids to cover the stress of the surgery and retest the pituitary adrenal access before stopping this.
- Have a careful anesthetic preoperative assessment with your anesthetic colleagues and ensure the patient is metabolically stable if possible through block and replacement treatment.

Pitfalls

- Be careful of missing subclinical Cushing's where the patient has no clinical features of the disease, but autonomous cortisol secretion is present enough to suppress the contralateral adrenal gland.
- Consent for the known potential complications.
- Do not fail to monitor postoperative electrolytes and risks of infection.
- Ensure good quality assistance and plenty of time – this is not an operation to do under avoidable pressure.
- Physical signs of complications such as infection (including temperature and typical leukocytosis and CRP estimations) can be totally missed and absent in patients with high cortisol levels.

Further Reading

Clutter WE. Cushing's syndrome; hypercortisolism. In: Doherty GM, Skogseid B, editors. Surgical endocrinology. Philadelphia: Lippincott Williams & Wilkins; 2001. p. 237.

Langer P, Cupisti K, Bartsch DK, et al. Adrenal involvement in MEN type 1. World J Surg. 2002;26(8):891–6.

Lezoche E, Guerrieri M, Feliciotti AM, et al. Anterior, lateral and posterior retroperitoneal approaches in endoscopic adrenalectomy. Surg Endosc. 2002;16(1):96–9.

Patel HRH, Harris AM, Lennard TWJ. Adrenal masses: the investigation and management of adrenal incidentalomas. Ann R Coll Surg Engl. 2001;83:250–2.

Stratakis CA, Boikas SA. Genetics of adrenal tumours associated with Cushing's Syndrome: a new classification for bilateral adrenocortical hyperplasias. Nat Clin Pract Endocrinol Metab. 2007;3(11):748–57.

Chapter 3
Management of Conn's Syndrome

Vasilis A. Constantinides and Fausto Palazzo

Definitions

Aldosterone Physiology and Its Dysregulation: Conn's Syndrome

- Aldosterone is the major mineralocorticoid steroid hormone. It is synthesized from cholesterol and secreted from the *zona glomerulosa* of the adrenal cortex.
- Major determinants of aldosterone secretion include the renin-angiotensin system (RAS) and the serum potassium (K^+) concentration.

  - Relative hypovolemia is detected by the juxtaglomerular apparatus of the nephron and results in renin secretion into the circulation.
  - Renin catalyzes the conversion of angiotensinogen to angiotensin I in the liver; this is in turn converted to angiotensin II via a proteolytic process catalyzed by the angiotensin-converting enzyme (ACE) in the lungs.
  - Angiotensin II and angiotensin III (its breakdown product) both have direct pressor effects on the vasculature but more importantly are potent stimulators of aldosterone secretion.

- Other additional lesser regulators of aldosterone production include:

  - Adrenocorticotrophic hormone (ACTH)
  - Atrial natriuretic peptide and dopamine (both inhibitory)
  - Hyperkalemia independently stimulates aldosterone secretion in the *zona glomerulosa*

V.A. Constantinides • F. Palazzo (✉)
Department of Thyroid and Endocrine Surgery,
Imperial College NHS Trust, Hammersmith Campus, London, UK
e-mail: f.palazzo@imperial.ac.uk

J.C. Watkinson, D.M. Scott-Coombes (eds.), *Tips and Tricks in Endocrine Surgery*,
DOI 10.1007/978-1-4471-2146-6_3, © Springer-Verlag London 2014

- Aldosterone's primary effect is uptake and retention of sodium with water via an active transport and osmotic mechanism, respectively, with potassium and hydrogen excretion accompanying the ion shifts. The target organs to achieve this are:
  - The distal convoluted tubule of the kidney
  - Gastrointestinal mucosa, salivary, and sweat glands

Aldosterone Excess (Hyperaldosteronism)

- Hyperaldosteronism has detrimental effects through a mechanism of oxidative stress and collagen remodelling. The end result includes endothelial dysfunction, left ventricular hypertrophy, and widespread organ fibrosis.
- The incidence of circulatory diseases (stroke, acute coronary syndromes) in patients with hyperaldosteronism is significantly higher compared to patients with essential hypertension, and mineralocorticoid antagonists decrease mortality in patients with heart failure.
- Hyperaldosteronism may be classified as primary or secondary depending on the underlying pathology.
- Primary aldosteronism (PA) was first described by Jerome Conn in 1955 in a young woman with an aldosterone-secreting adrenal adenoma.
- Several other causes of PA have since been identified (Table 3.1) with bilateral adrenal hyperplasia responsible for around 60 % of cases.
- Secondary hyperaldosteronism results from excessive activation of the RAS without a primary disorder of the *zona glomerulosa* itself (Table 3.1).

Epidemiology of Conn's Syndrome

- Incidence is unknown.
- Prevalence of 3.4–11.2 % has been demonstrated in hospital-treated patients with essential hypertension.
- Up to 19 % of patients hospitalized for the treatment of their hypertension have primary hyperaldosteronism.
- The prevalence of the disease increases with the severity of the hypertension.
- Affects young adults between 30 and 50 years of age.
- Female to male ratio 3:1.
- No specific ethnic distribution.

Presentation (See Chap. 1)

- Typical early presentation with moderate hypertension
- Hypokalemia.

Table 3.1 Causes and subtypes of primary and secondary hyperaldosteronism

Causes of primary hyperaldosteronism	Percentage of cases	Remarks
Aldosterone-producing adenoma (APA)	~35 %	Original pathology described by Conn
Bilateral idiopathic adrenal hyperplasia (BAH)	~60 %	–
Primary unilateral adrenal hyperplasia	2 %	–
Pure aldosterone-producing adrenocortical carcinoma	<1 %	–
Familial aldosteronism (FH-I and FH-II)		AD, fusion of ACTH-responsive 11-beta-hydroxylase gene promoter to aldosterone synthase gene
1. Type I – glucocorticoid remediable	<1 %	
2. Type II – familial aldosteronoma or hyperplasia	<2 %	
Ectopic aldosterone-producing adenoma/carcinoma	<0.1 %	Ovarian and renal tumors
Causes of secondary hyperaldosteronism		
Disorders of edema		
1. Cardiac failure		
2. Liver failure/cirrhosis		
3. Nephrotic syndrome		
States of reduced renal perfusion		
1. Renal artery stenosis		
2. Advanced atherosclerosis		
3. Malignant hypertension		
Renin-producing tumors		
Pregnancy		

AD autosomal dominant, *ACTH* adrenocorticotrophic hormone

- Normokalemia occurs in up to 50 % of patients and, therefore, does not reliably exclude the need to screen for PA.
- Hypernatremia (serum Na$^+$ >145 mmol/l) without peripheral edema.
- Alkalosis.
- Symptoms from aldosterone-induced organ damage such acute coronary syndromes, stroke, obesity, and insulin resistance/diabetes mellitus.

Indications for screening for PA in a hypertensive patient include:

- Early onset (<20 years)
- Resistance to two or more medications
- Severe hypertension (systolic blood pressure >160 or diastolic blood pressure >100 mmHg)
- Hypertension with spontaneous hypokalemia (or secondary to low-dose diuretic)
- Hypertension associated with an adrenal incidentaloma
- Evaluation for secondary causes of hypertension
- Family history of hypertension and PA

Diagnostic Evaluation

- Accurate diagnosis depends on biochemical tests and radiological investigations.
- Liaise with endocrinologists.

Basic Biochemical Tests: (See Chap. 1)

- Plasma aldosterone concentration (PAC, pmol/L)
- Plasma renin activity (PRA, pmol/ml/hour)
- Active renin concentration (ARC, pmol/ml/hour)
- PAC: PRA ratio
- Hypertension during the period off these drugs can be managed with alpha-adrenergic and non-dihydropyridine calcium channel blockade with medication such as doxazosin and diltiazem together with potassium supplements.
- The PAC: PRA ratio is a screening test with variable diagnostic accuracy and a sensitivity and specificity of between 64–100 % and 87–100 %.
- Patients meeting the diagnostic criteria for PA based on a positive PAC: PRA test should undergo confirmatory testing before a definitive diagnosis of primary aldosteronism is made.

Confirmatory Testing

Suppression of aldosterone production after expansion of intravascular volume is the pathophysiological basis of most confirmatory testing. A positive test is characterized by a paradoxical unsuppressable aldosterone level. Three tests have been employed:

Saline Suppression Test (SST)

- The most widely performed test.
- After stopping all interfering drugs as above and a low-sodium diet for 3 days, 2 l of normal saline are given intravenously over 4 h.
- Measurement of plasma aldosterone and urinary aldosterone and sodium levels at the 4 h time point.
- A PAC level of >10 pmol/L, urinary aldosterone secretion >12 ug/24 h, and with urinary sodium >200 mmol/24 h confirm the diagnosis of PA.
- This test is contraindicated in patients with severe uncontrolled hypertension, renal and cardiac failure, arrhythmia, or severe hypokalemia.

Fludrocortisone Suppression Test (FST)

- Now infrequently used because it requires hospitalization, may be associated with severe hypokalemia and deterioration in cardiac function.

Captopril Suppression Test (CST)

- Now infrequently used also due to false-negative rates of up to 36 %.

Lateralization Studies

The therapeutic pathway of the patient depends on whether the cause of the hyperaldosteronism is unilateral or bilateral. All patients with positive biochemical testing require a dedicated, high-resolution computed tomography (CT) scan of the adrenal glands with thin collimation (2–3 mm slices). Possible findings on CT may include:

- Normal-appearing adrenal glands
- Solitary, unilateral, hypodense (≤10 Hounsfield units) adenoma with normal contralateral adrenal gland
- Minimal unilateral adrenal limb thickening
- Bilateral nodularity

As 95 % of PA is caused by either BAH or APA, any test used for subtype evaluation needs to be able to reliably distinguish between these two pathologies since their treatment differs significantly.

- CT alone is insufficiently sensitive ranging between 58 and 75 %.
- Fewer than 25 % of microadenomas (<1 cm in diameter) may be detected on CT scanning. Over half of patients with CT-detected unilateral microadenomas have the contralateral adrenal as the main source of aldosterone hypersecretion and 40 % of patients hypersecreting aldosterone unilaterally had normal CT findings.
- The principle cause of the inaccuracy is the 2–10 % chance of detecting a nonfunctioning "incidentaloma" and erroneously attributing this as the cause of the aldosterone excess.
- Magnetic resonance (MRI) imaging shares the same diagnostic accuracy as CT and should be reserved for patients with contraindications to the use of contrast.

In view of the above, patients who are potential surgical candidates require another test to reliably determine lateralization. The most popular and reliable test is adrenal venous sampling (AVS).

- While a very operator-dependant procedure, in experienced hands AVS is associated with success rates of up to 96 % and sensitivity and specificity for detecting unilateral hyperaldosteronism of 95 and 100 %, respectively.

Table 3.2 Treatment modalities for different types of primary aldosteronism

Medical management
Bilateral idiopathic adrenal hyperplasia (BAH)
Familial hyperaldosteronism type I
Patients who decline or are not candidates for surgery
Surgical management
Aldosterone-producing adenoma (APA)
Pure or mixed aldosterone-producing adrenocortical carcinoma
Primary unilateral adrenal hyperplasia
Familial aldosteronism type II
Ectopic aldosterone-producing adenoma/carcinoma

- The test involves femoral vein catheterization and the sampling of blood for aldosterone and cortisol levels (with or without prior synthetic ACTH stimulation) from the right and left adrenal veins, the inferior vena cava, and peripheral blood.
- Complication rates can be as low as 2.5 % and include adrenal necrosis, hemorrhage, anaphylaxis due to contrast administration, and venous thrombosis.
- A "cortisol-corrected aldosterone ratio" is used to compare each sampling site since it allows compensation for dilutional effects. An aldosterone to cortisol ratio of one adrenal vein versus the other of 4:1 is diagnostic of unilateral PA, and a ratio of <3:1 is indicative of bilateral PA.

A new lateralization modality is metomidate PET scanning that has produced very encouraging initial results and may limit the need for AVS in the future.

Genetic testing should be considered in patients with confirmed PA with particularly early onset (diagnosis before 20 years), especially in the presence of a positive family history of hypertension or stroke at a young age since familial hyperaldosteronism type I or FH-II may have implications both for the patient and other family members.

Treatment

The aim of treatment of PA is to control the hypertension, improve serum potassium concentration, and prevent morbidity from the direct deleterious effect of high aldosterone concentrations on the circulation and its end organs.

Medical Therapy (Indications Shown in Table 3.2)

This is delivered via a mineralocorticoid receptor antagonist (MRA) or in the case of rare variants, such as FH-I, with exogenous administration of steroids.

- The MRA most commonly used is spironolactone with a more recent drug eplerenone as the alternative.
- Spironolactone is a competitive MRA with affinity to androgen and progesterone receptors.

- Use may be limited (mainly in men) by dose-dependent side effects such as gynecomastia, decreased libido, and sexual dysfunction in up to 52 % of treated men. Menstrual irregularities and breast tenderness may occur in women as well as generalized gastrointestinal disturbances in both sexes.
- Eplerenone is a highly selective MRA with an affinity to sex hormone receptors that is 500-fold less than spironolactone.
- While the antihypertensive effects may be marginally inferior to spironolactone in patients with BAH, the side-effect profile is considerably more favorable.
- Eplerenone is five times more expensive than spironolactone so currently spironolactone is used as the first-line medical treatment, reserving eplerenone mainly for men suffering from unacceptable side effects.
- Glucocorticoids such as dexamethasone are used to treat glucocorticoid remediable aldosteronism (FH-I) by suppressing ACTH production. The lowest dexamethasone dose that is effective is used to avoid iatrogenic Cushing's syndrome.
- Other antihypertensive agents such as thiazide diuretics may be required in addition to a MRA to achieve optimal blood pressure control.

Surgical Management (Indications Shown in Table 3.2)

Minimally invasive adrenalectomy either via a transabdominal laparoscopic or a retroperitoneoscopic route is the optimal treatment for patients with APA, unilateral hyperplasia, and FH-2. Open adrenalectomy is still currently recommended in patients with suspected adrenocortical carcinoma or with tumors where a minimally invasive approach is not an option.

Preoperative General Considerations

- Preoperative control of hypertension is essential for safe surgery and usually requires appropriate expertise and multiple medications.
- Correction of hypokalemia with potassium replacement and treatment with a MRA is necessary preoperatively to minimize risks of cardiac arrhythmias.
- Attention is required to detect possible effects of aldosterone excess to the coronary circulation as well as subclinical diabetes mellitus.

Postoperative General Considerations

- PAC can be measured on the first postoperative day to confirm surgical cure.
- Urea and electrolytes are monitored and plasma potassium concentration corrected. Potassium supplementation can usually be withdrawn within 48 h (not always immediately due to compensation for intracellular potassium deficit).
- Spironolactone may be stopped postoperatively, and other antihypertensive medication may be reduced or stopped completely, depending on local policies.

Table 3.3 The aldosteronoma resolution score to measure the likelihood of complete cure from hypertension postoperatively

Variables		
Need for ≤2 antihypertensive medication		
BMI <25 kg/m^2		
<6 months hypertension duration		
Female gender		
Likelihood level	**Number of variables**	**Accuracy** (%)
Low	0–1	27
Medium	2–3	46
High	4	75

BMI body mass index

Outcomes

- Approximately 90 % of patients that undergo an adrenalectomy for a unilateral adrenal adenoma secreting aldosterone reap benefit from their surgery. Approximately 40 % of patients remain hypertensive but are able to reduce their medication requirement. The remaining 50 % are able to stop all medication. The success is tightly linked to the length of the history of hypertension since irreversible cardiovascular changes are known to occur with time.
- The aldosteronoma resolution score (ARS) may aid in predicting complete resolution of hypertension based on four variables and three likelihood levels (Table 3.3).

Pearls and Pitfalls

Pearls	Pitfalls
Consider PA in the differential diagnosis of any young patient with hypertension +/− hypokalemia	Medication may affect screening results for PA
Adrenal venous sampling is recommended in all patients considered for adrenalectomy	Poor preoperative localization may lead to misguided surgery
Vigilant postoperative monitoring is necessary to correct hyperkalemia and hypotension at their onset	Insufficient patient counselling as to the likelihood of postoperative resolution of hypertension
Retroperitoneoscopic/laparoscopic adrenalectomy by a surgeon experienced in the technique may be the treatment of choice for unilateral PA	Partial adrenalectomy may fail to cure as APAs may be small and multiple

Additional factors associated with postoperative normotension include the lack of family history of hypertension, young age, positive response to spironolactone, and a high preoperative PAC: PRA ratio.

Further Reading

Burton TJ, Mackenzie IS, Balan K, et al. Evaluation of the sensitivity and specificity of 11C-metomidate positron emission tomography (PET)-CT for lateralizing aldosterone secretion by Conn's adenomas. J Clin Endocrinol Metab. 2012;97(1):100–9.

Conn JW. Presidential address. I. Painting background. II. Primary aldosteronism, a new clinical syndrome. J Lab Clin Med. 1955;45(1):3–17.

Gallay BJ, Ahmad S, Xu L, et al. Screening for primary aldosteronism without discontinuing hypertensive medications: plasma aldosterone-renin ratio. Am J Kidney Dis. 2001;37(4):699–705.

Giacchetti G, Ronconi V, Lucarelli G, et al. Analysis of screening and confirmatory tests in the diagnosis of primary aldosteronism: need for a standardized protocol. J Hypertens. 2006;24(4):737–45.

Mattsson C, Young Jr WF. Primary aldosteronism: diagnostic and treatment strategies. Nat Clin Pract Nephrol. 2006;2(4):198–208; quiz, 1 p following 30.

Milliez P, Girerd X, Plouin PF, et al. Evidence for an increased rate of cardiovascular events in patients with primary aldosteronism. J Am Coll Cardiol. 2005;45(8):1243–8.

Montori VM, Young Jr WF. Use of plasma aldosterone concentration-to-plasma renin activity ratio as a screening test for primary aldosteronism. A systematic review of the literature. Endocrinol Metab Clin North Am. 2002;31(3):619–32, xi.

Rossi GP, Bernini G, Caliumi C, et al. A prospective study of the prevalence of primary aldosteronism in 1,125 hypertensive patients. J Am Coll Cardiol. 2006;48(11):2293–300.

Schwartz GL, Turner ST. Screening for primary aldosteronism in essential hypertension: diagnostic accuracy of the ratio of plasma aldosterone concentration to plasma renin activity. Clin Chem. 2005;51(2):386–94.

Young WF, Stanson AW, Thompson GB, et al. Role for adrenal venous sampling in primary aldosteronism. Surgery. 2004;136(6):1227–35.

Chapter 4
Pheochromocytoma and Paraganglioma

Michael J. Stechman

Definition

- Pheochromocytoma (PHEO) and paraganglioma (PGL) are rare tumors that secrete catecholamines and their metabolites.
- PHEOs arise from the autonomic neuroendocrine tissue of the adrenal medulla.
- PGLs develop in extra-adrenal autonomic neuroendocrine tissue: those derived from extra-adrenal sympathetics may occur anywhere along the sympathetic chain (in decreasing order of incidence: juxtarenal, para-aortic, bladder, thoracic). Head and neck PGL are usually nonfunctioning tumors derived from the parasympathetic nervous system.
- Tumors usually secrete either predominantly noradrenaline or noradrenaline and adrenaline and may be classed as noradrenergic or adrenergic tumors, respectively.

Epidemiology and Pathology

- PHEO (85–90 % of tumors) and PGL (10–15 %) are uncommon and have an incidence of 1–4 cases per 100,000 of population annually.
- Male to female ratio is 1:1.
- Approximately 70 % of tumors are sporadic and their etiology is unknown. The remainder are genetic in origin.
- Median age of diagnosis is 55 years in sporadic cases but lower in those of genetic origin (approximately 70 % diagnosed within first two decades of life).

M.J. Stechman, MB, ChB, MD
Department of Endocrine Surgery,
University Hospital of Wales, Heath Park,
Cardiff, CF 14 4XW, UK
e-mail: michael.stechman@wales.nhs.uk

J.C. Watkinson, D.M. Scott-Coombes (eds.), *Tips and Tricks in Endocrine Surgery*,
DOI 10.1007/978-1-4471-2146-6_4, © Springer-Verlag London 2014

Table 4.1 Familial disorders which are associated with the development of PHEO and/or PGL

Syndrome	Gene (chromosome)[a,b]	Clinical manifestations	% With PHEO	% Bilateral
von Hippel-Lindau[c]	*VHL* (3p25-p26)	PHEO, cerebellar hemangioblastoma, retinal angiomas, renal cell carcinoma, pancreatic cysts, pancreatic NETs in 5–10 %	10–20 %	40–80
Multiple endocrine neoplasia type 2A[d]	*RET* (10q11.2)	PHEO, MTC, hyperparathyroidism	50 %	50–80
Multiple endocrine neoplasia type 2B		PHEO, MTC, mucosal neuromas, colonic ganglioneuromatosis, marfanoid facies, skeletal abnormalities		
von Recklinghausen's disease	*NF1* (17q11.2)	Neurofibromata, >6 café au lait spots, axillary freckling, skeletal abnormalities, and PHEO	5–10 %	10
PGL-1	*SDHD* (11q23)	Parasympathetic head and neck PGL +/– PHEO	Uncommon	–
PGL-2	*SDHAF2* (11q13.1)	Parasympathetic head and neck PGL (nonfunctioning)	Not described	–
PGL-3	*SDHC* (1q21)	Parasympathetic head and neck PGL, PHEO rare	Rare	–
PGL-4	*SDHB* (1p35-p36)	Sympathetic abdominal PGL and PHEO – 50 % malignant	PGL or PHEO in 70 %	
Familial pheochromocytoma	*TMEM127* (2q11)	PHEO	?	43
Familial neural crest-derived tumors	*KIF1B* (1p36.2)	PHEO or neuroblastoma	?	?

[a]*RET* rearranged during transfection, *SDH* succinate dehydrogenase, *SDHAF2* succinate dehydrogenase complex assembly factor 2, *TMEM127* transmembrane 127, *NF1* neurofibromatosis type 1, *KIF1B* kinesin family member 1B (microtubule motor)
[b]Homozygous mutations of *SDHA* cause Leigh syndrome which is not associated with PHEO or PGL
[c]Four types of VHL disease are recognized (1, 2A, 2B, and 2C) – type 1 is not associated with PHEO
[d]Medullary thyroid cancer (MTC) is usually the initial presentation. MEN2A is associated with Hirschsprung's disease in 5%
? not currently known

- The genetic disorders multiple endocrine neoplasia type 2 (MEN2), von Hippel-Lindau disease (VHL), neurofibromatosis type 1 (NF1), and the inherited paraganglioma syndromes (PGL-1,-3, and -4) are all associated with significantly increased risk of the development of PHEO or PGL (Table 4.1).
- PHEO/PGL of genetic origin is more likely to be bilateral, extra-adrenal, multifocal and associated with an increased risk of malignancy.

- Macroscopically, PHEO and PGL are soft vascular tumors with a pink-tan color on slicing. Microscopically, they exhibit a regular nested "Zellballen" pattern of polyhedral cells that are chromaffin positive on staining.
- The definitive markers for malignancy are local invasion and distant metastasis. However size >5 cm, presence of lymphovascular or capsular invasion, and increased Ki-67 proliferation index are associated with increased risk.

Presentation

- May be symptomatic or asymptomatic.
- Symptomatic tumors present with typical triad of paroxysmal headache (90 %), sweating (92 %), and palpitations (72 %).
- 0.2 % of patients investigated for hypertension will have a PHEO, and 70 % of those with PHEO will have sustained hypertension.
- About 10 % of PHEO are discovered incidentally on CT/MRI for unrelated symptoms (adrenal "incidentaloma").
- Asymptomatic tumors may be diagnosed during screening for genetic disorders in which PHEO or PGL is part of the disease phenotype (in order of commonality, VHL, MEN2A or B, NF1, SDHB/C/D).
- Clinical signs are usually absent.

Investigations (See Chap. 1)

- The diagnosis is biochemical.
- Measure plasma or urinary metanephrines.
- Metanephrine and/or catecholamine values that are 4 times greater than upper limit of normal are 100 % diagnostic for functioning PHEO and PGL.
- Sympathomimetics and other drugs should be stopped prior to testing.
- Positive biochemical testing should be followed by cross-sectional adrenal imaging since this is the most common location.
- Abdominopelvic computed tomography (CT) or magnetic resonance imaging (MRI) have a sensitivity of 90–100 % and a specificity of 70–80 %, especially if tumor size is >1 cm (Fig. 4.1). In individuals with inherited paraganglioma syndromes, USS is useful for neck surveillance (*SDHC* and *D* mutations). Extra-adrenal lesions may occur anywhere along the sympathetic chain and will require detailed examination CT or MRI of the chest, abdomen, and pelvis.
- Functional imaging with ^{123}I-labeled metaiodobenzylguanidine (^{123}I-MIBG) is not necessary for the majority of adrenal tumors but may be useful in patients with extra-adrenal masses or those with genetic disease owing to the higher incidence of multifocal, bilateral, and malignant disease (Fig. 4.2).
- Some forms of positron emission tomography (PET), e.g., ^{18}F-fluorodopamine PET, are more sensitive than ^{123}I-MIBG but are not widely available. This should

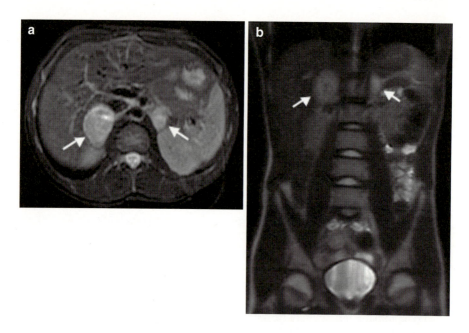

Fig. 4.1 Axial (**a**) and coronal (**b**) images from the MRI abdomen of a 13 year old boy with VHL disease. Bilateral PHEO were diagnosed on biochemical screening. Note the hyperintense appearance of the tumours (*white arrows*) on axial T2 weighted images

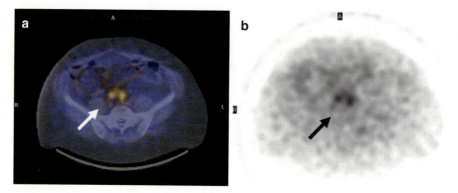

Fig. 4.2 Axial fused SPECT CT and ^{123}I-MIBG (**a**) and planar ^{123}I-MIBG images (**b**) in a 50 year old patient with SDHB disease and recurrent PGL just below the aortic bifurcation (*white and black arrows*)

be reserved for patients with biochemical evidence of disease and negative localization by usual modalities.

• Selective adrenal vein sampling has no role for PHEO.

Medical Management

- Multidisciplinary approach between an experienced endocrinologist, radiologist, and surgeon is vital in managing such patients.
- Diagnosis of PHEO or PGL should be followed by initiation of pharmacological alpha-adrenergic receptor blockade and prompt surgical excision.
- The target blood pressure is less than 120/80 mmHg with a significant postural drop on standing (>10 mmHg drop in systolic blood pressure)
- Several regimens are described:
  - Oral alpha-adrenergic blockers (phenoxybenzamine, doxazosin, or prazosin, given orally for at least 14 days preoperatively).
  - Oral calcium channel blockers (nicardipine, as an infusion intraoperatively).
  - Oral metyrosine (catecholamine synthesis blocker) may be helpful in the presence of cardiac failure.
- Beta-adrenergic blockade to control tachycardia (e.g., oral propranolol) should be commenced only after adequate alpha-blockade to prevent dangerous hypertension that arises with unopposed alpha-induced vasoconstriction.

Indications for Surgery

- Following medical preparation, excision of the PHEO or PGL is indicated in all patients that are fit for surgery.
- Rare cases presenting with metastatic disease often benefit from debulking or excision of the primary tumor to improve symptom control and response to adjuvant therapy (radioactive ^{131}I-MIBG, chemotherapy, or tyrosine kinase inhibitors).
- A minority of patients present with cardiac failure or myocardial ischemia and rapid surgical treatment following alpha-blockade may be lifesaving in such cases.

Tips for Surgery

Preoperative

- Ensure satisfactory pharmacological blockade prior to surgery.
- Check the anatomical site of the tumor on recent cross-sectional imaging.
- For larger tumors, look for signs of metastatic disease or local invasion that would alter operative approach.

Operative

- For adrenal tumors, the best approach is laparoscopic or retroperitoneoscopic, even for large cystic tumors (>10 cm), provided there are no signs of local invasion on preoperative imaging.
- For juxta-renal and other extra-adrenal abdominal or thoracic tumors – laparotomy/thoracotomy and open excision is favored because:
  - Proximity of visceral/great vessels may render minimally invasive treatment unfeasible.
  - Increased risk of malignancy and local recurrence.

- In patients with evidence of malignant disease, open surgery and en bloc excision of the tumor with involved structures is the most appropriate approach.
- These tumors are highly vascular and liable to capsular rupture (which may predispose to local recurrence) if not handled with caution.
- Poor laparoscopic views can sometimes be improved by use of tonsillar swabs to absorb blood and decrease light absorption in the operative field.
- Use of energy devices (bipolar diathermy, ultrasonic dissector) may be less effective due to development of fragile neovascular vessels over the tumor. In such cases endoscopic ligation clips may be helpful.

Postoperative

- Some patients may require level 3 care for short-term vasopressor treatment for hypotension secondary to alpha-blockade.
- However, recovery is rapid in most patients, especially when endoscopic techniques are employed.
- Blood glucose levels must be regularly monitored as patients may rarely develop hypoglycemia.
- Patients under the age of 50 years with PHEO should be counselled for genetic testing (in the following order: VHL, RET and SDHB, and D). Those with PGL should undergo SDHB, C, and D testing.

Complications and Outcomes

- The BAETS national endocrine audit database reports that the overall mortality from adrenal surgery is <1 % and the mean length of stay for laparoscopic adrenalectomy is 4.2 days versus 9.5 days for open adrenalectomy. The majority of patients recover fully from surgery, and recurrent disease is very rare. A summary of complications is given in Table 4.2.

Table 4.2 Complications of surgical excision of functioning PHEO or PGL

Immediate	Early	Late
Bleeding – ICV or left renal vein. May require conversion to open surgery	Hypotension secondary to alpha-blockade	Port site or incisional hernia
Hemodynamic instability – hypertensive stroke or MI, arrhythmia, cardiac arrest	Ileus, respiratory or urinary tract infection, thromboembolic event	Local or distant recurrence due to undiagnosed malignant disease
Thermal injury to adjacent bowel, blood vessels, or organs, e.g., spleen	Addisonian crisis – bilateral or subtotal adrenalectomy	Addisonian crisis in steroid dependent patients
	Continued bleeding – rare	

Malignant or Metastatic Disease

- Surgery with curative intent or cytoreductive procedures offers the best treatment for those with malignant disease, and the latter may improve the efficacy of adjuvant treatment:

  - Radioactive ^{131}I-MIBG – 60 % of metastases exhibit uptake, and tumor response is seen in 30 %, while 40–50 % will show disease stabilization.
  - Radioactive ^{111}In-pentetreotide and ^{111}I-DOTA-octreotide – these compounds may be of use in those with octreotide scintigraphy-positive disease. However, it is less effective than radioactive MIBG.
  - Other therapies – cyclophosphamide, vincristine, and dacarbazine (CVD) combination chemotherapy may improve symptoms in 50 % of patients but does not improve survival. Trials of the tyrosine kinase inhibitor sunitinib have demonstrated a partial response in a small number of patients.

Pearls and Pitfalls

- MDT management involving individuals with experience in treating PHEO/PGL is essential.
- Diagnosis of PHEO/PGL is biochemical – equivocal biochemical results should be followed by retesting.
- For those with convincing biochemistry and an isolated adrenal mass, functional imaging rarely adds anything to the management.
- All patients with PGL and those below the age of 50 years with PHEO should be referred for genetic testing.
- Follow-up should be lifelong to detect late recurrence, since malignant behavior is difficult to predict.
- Bilateral disease may be treated with subtotal adrenalectomy if one or both of the tumors are less than 2.5 cm in size in VHL but not in MEN2-related disease (increased risk of recurrence due to background adrenal medullary hyperplasia).
- Such patients should be tested for steroid insufficiency prior to discharge (short synacthen test).

Further Reading

Chrisoulidou A, Kaltsas G, Ilias I, Grossman AB. The diagnosis and management of malignant phaeochromocytoma and paraganglioma. Endocr Relat Cancer. 2007;14(3):569–85.

Erlic Z, Neumann HP. When should genetic testing be obtained in a patient with phaeochromocytoma or paraganglioma? Clin Endocrinol (Oxf). 2009;70(3):354–7.

Gagner M, Lacroix A, Bolte E. Laparoscopic adrenalectomy in Cushing's syndrome and pheochromocytoma. N Engl J Med. 1992;327(14):1033.

Lenders JW, Pacak K, Walther MM, Linehan WM, Mannelli M, Friberg P, Keiser HR, Goldstein DS, Eisenhofer G. Biochemical diagnosis of pheochromocytoma: which test is best? JAMA. 2002;287(11):1427–34.

Walz MK, Alesina PF, Wenger FA, Koch JA, Neumann HP, Petersenn S, Schmid KW, Mann K. Laparoscopic and retroperitoneoscopic treatment of pheochromocytomas and retroperitoneal paragangliomas: results of 161 tumors in 126 patients. World J Surg. 2006;30(5):899–908.

Chapter 5
Adrenocortical Carcinoma and Open Adrenalectomy

Radu Mihai

Definition and Staging

In the absence of metastases (stage IV disease) or local invasion into surrounding viscera (stage III), the diagnosis of adrenocortical carcinoma (ACC) in adrenal tumors >5 cm (stage II) or <5 cm (stage I disease) remains very challenging.

Incidence

ACC is one of the rarest tumors, with an incidence of ≈1–3 case/million population and two peaks in childhood and at 50–70 years. In the UK, some 150 cases are diagnosed yearly.

Symptoms

Nonfunctional tumors are found incidentally on scans performed for unrelated complaints or present with signs of local compression due to their large volume. Functional tumors present with rapid onset of gross clinical signs and/or symptoms of Cushing's syndrome. Virilization of female patients and feminization of male patients (e.g., gynecomastia) are very suggestive of malignant tumors.

R. Mihai, MD, PhD, FRCS
Department of Endocrine Surgery,
John Radcliffe Hospital, Headley Way,
Oxford OX3 9DU, UK
e-mail: r_mihai99@hotmail.com

J.C. Watkinson, D.M. Scott-Coombes (eds.), *Tips and Tricks in Endocrine Surgery*,
DOI 10.1007/978-1-4471-2146-6_5, © Springer-Verlag London 2014

Preoperative Assessment

Biochemical Assessment

- Pheochromocytoma should be excluded by measuring 24-h urinary metanephrines.
- An overnight dexamethasone test (1 mg dexamethasone (DXM) administered orally at 23:00 before collecting blood for serum cortisol the following morning at 08:00) is a reliable screening test for Cushing's syndrome. If this screening test is positive (i.e., if cortisol >100 nmol/l the morning after DXM), the ACTH-independent Cushing's syndrome is confirmed by proving plasma ACTH is suppressed and that 24-h urinary excretion is not inhibited by high-dose steroids (DXM 2 ms qds for 2 days).
- In hypertensive patients, the aldosterone/renin ratio should assess for primary hyperaldosteronism.
- Plasma levels of androstenedione, DHEAS (dihydroepiandrostenedione sulfate), 17-OH progesterone, testosterone, and estradiol will characterize the secretion of androgen precursors.
- Very recently it has been shown that the urinary excretion of steroid precursors has a very specific "signature" for malignancy.

Radiological Assessment

CT scans demonstrate an inhomogenous irregular mass with high intensity on enhanced images (>20 Hounsfield units) and rapid washout of contrast. CT also provides anatomical details of the possible involvement of surrounding viscera (liver/pancreas/kidney) and can demonstrate liver/lung metastases.

PET scan is done to assess for metastatic disease and to characterize the tumor (standardized uptake value (SUV) >40 or SUV 1.5 higher than liver are highly characteristic for malignant tumors).

Laparoscopic Adrenalectomy: No Role in Patients with Known or Suspected ACC

Though several series have reported successful laparoscopic excision of ACCs <8 cm, the view held by most experts is that surgical treatment for ACC involves radical local excision that cannot be secured via a laparoscopic approach.

Informed Consent

The preoperative imaging should allow the surgeon to predict whether the operation will also include nephrectomy, splenectomy, distal pancreatectomy, or inferior vena cava (IVC) venotomy (for controlling IVC thrombus), and the consent should include appropriate information about the risk associated with such associated interventions.

Perioperative Management

DVT prophylaxis should be instituted (intraoperative use of mechanical compression followed postoperatively by Fragmin®/thromboembolic deterrent stockings).

Antibiotic prophylaxis is routinely used in patients with Cushing's syndrome but could be omitted in patients with nonsecreting tumors.

Intravenous steroids should be given preoperatively (100 mg hydrocortisone) and be continued until oral steroid can be tolerated.

Radical Adrenalectomy for ACC

The aim of the operation is to remove the tumor in continuity with viscera that could be invaded "en bloc" which should increase the likelihood of achieving negative resection margins (R0 resection).

How to Perform a Right Open Adrenalectomy for ACC

- *Incision*. A rooftop incision extending towards the right flank and crossing the midline offers best access.
- *Mobilizing the Right Kidney*. With the exception of small tumors that can be easily dissected off the upper pole of the right kidney, ACC should be excised in continuity with the kidney and perinephric fat within the Gerota's fascia. The hepatic flexure is mobilized fully. Duodenum is kocherized to allow exposure of the IVC. The retroperitoneal space is dissected from lateral to medial, starting at the lower pole of the kidney. The right ureter is identified, tied, and divided. The right gonadal vessels should be identified and protected up to the drainage point into the IVC. The renal vessels are ligated and divided. A sling should be passed around the IVC if clamping the IVC later in the procedure is anticipated.

- *Mobilizing the Liver*. If there is suspicion of IVC invasion, one needs to secure control of the IVC at the subdiaphragmatic level. The lateral triangular ligament is divided; the bare area of the liver is exposed, mobilizing the diaphragm. The right triangular ligament is divided. Careful dissection close to the crus of the diaphragm allows the IVC to be slinged and prepared for later clamping, if needed.
- *Dissection of the IVC*. From the infrarenal IVC exposed earlier, the dissection progresses proximally aiming to create a "groove" between the tumor and the IVC. Care should be shown close to subhepatic vessels.
- *Dissection of the Right Lobe of the Liver*. One needs to assess if there is a dissection plane that would allow mobilization of the tumor without breaching its capsule. If there is direct invasion into the liver, one needs to ask support from a liver surgeon who could assist in performing a limited right hepatectomy in continuity with the tumor.

How to Perform a Left Open Adrenalectomy for ACC

- *Incision*. A rooftop incision extending towards the left flank and crossing the midline offers best access.
- *Mobilizing the Left Colon*. The splenic flexure is fully mobilized, the peritoneal reflection along the descending colon divided, the gastrocolic ligament divided, and the entire left colon mobilized distally. Care should be shown to avoid injury to the mesocolon and main arterial and venous branches. Once the mesocolon is fully mobilized, the fourth part of duodenum becomes visible (Treitz angle).
- *Mobilizing the Left Kidney*. The retroperitoneal space is dissected from lateral to medial, starting at the lower pole of the kidney. The left ureter is identified, tied, and divided. The gonadal vessels should be identified, tied, and divided distal from their drainage point into left renal vein.
- *Management of the Pancreas*. In the presence of a large left adrenal tumor, the tail of the pancreas is "stretched" over the tumor, and a distal pancreatectomy is likely to provide safer oncological procedure. After identifying the inferior mesenteric vein (IMV), a tunnel is created under the body of the pancreas to the left of IMV, and the body of the pancreas is transected using a linear stapler. The resection line is usually sutured. A Robinson drain is placed next to the pancreatic bed as a pancreatic fistula is a common postoperative complication.
- *Management of the Spleen*. If the splenic artery is seen on preoperative CT scans to be surrounded or displaced by the tumor, it is safer (and easier) to perform a simultaneous splenectomy. The splenic artery/vein should be identified at the upper border of the body of the pancreas, ligated, and divided.

Histological Assessment

Histological criteria for the diagnosis of ACC are summarized by the *Weiss score* (Table 5.1), and the diagnosis of ACC is suspected when the score is >3 and confirmed when the score is >6.

Table 5.1 Histological appearance associated with adrenocortical cancer

Histological criteria assessed for the Weiss score
High mitotic rate
Atypical mitoses
High nuclear grade
Low percentage of clear cells
Necrosis
Diffuse architecture of tumor
Capsular invasion
Sinusoidal invasion
Venous invasion

Postoperative Care

Steroid Replacement. Intravenous steroids (100 mg hydrocortisone IV qds) are maintained until diet is restarted and then converted to oral steroids (hydrocortisone, 20–20–10 mg/day, aiming to decrease by 5 mg/day every 3–5 days).

DVT prophylaxis continues during the admission, in parallel with early mobilization.

Oral intake can be resumed within 24 h postoperatively.

Management of Patients with Localized ACC

If there is no radiological evidence of distant metastases, it remains debatable if patients need adjuvant Mitotane® chemotherapy. The *European Network of the Study of Adrenal Tumors* (ENSAT) is due to initiate a multicenter randomized trial that will investigate whether Mitotane® improves disease-free and overall survival benefits.

Pearls

- Feasibility of resection is determined by invasion of IVC (right) or superior mesenteric artery (left).
- Aim for R0 Resection
- Tumors of indeterminate malignancy can be approached with a trial laparoscopic dissection.

Pitfalls

- Laparoscopic surgery has no role for clearly malignant tumors.
- All patients should undergo a postoperative synacthen test, even if there was no preoperative suspicion of Cushing's syndrome.
- Adrenocortical carcinoma should be managed in centers with a large experience of adrenal and endocrine surgery.

Chapter 6
Adrenal Metastasectomy

Gregory P. Sadler

Introduction

Metastasis to the adrenal gland from primary cancers is not uncommon and is usually indicative of widespread incurable metastatic disease. Cancers that commonly metastasize to the adrenal include:

- Lung
- Renal cell
- Colon
- Prostate
- Breast

Isolated adrenal metastasis with no evidence of other spread is rare. When identified however, these lesions may be considered suitable for resection if the clinical circumstances support this action. Cancers that appear to result in isolated adrenal metastasis include (in frequency of occurrence):

- Renal cell
- Colorectal
- Lung

Resection of true isolated metastasis has been demonstrated to increase survival in some patients and may occasionally be regarded as a curative in a very small number of patients, particularly those with renal cell cancer. Clearly this is not an area where a randomized trial is likely, and so each case must be evaluated on individual merits.

G.P. Sadler, MD, FRCS Gen Surg (Eng)
Department of Endocrine Surgery,
John Radcliffe Hospital, Headley Way,
Headington, Oxford OX3 9DU, UK
e-mail: gregsadler@btinternet.com

J.C. Watkinson, D.M. Scott-Coombes (eds.), *Tips and Tricks in Endocrine Surgery*,
DOI 10.1007/978-1-4471-2146-6_6, © Springer-Verlag London 2014

Lesions should be removed with minimum morbidity and mortality. Laparoscopic resection is the preferred surgical procedure when indicated, though may not always be possible. Experience has shown that these lesions are often locally infiltrative and can on occasion be difficult to resect. They are best referred to a specialist unit experienced in adrenal surgery.

Algorithm for Selection of Patients for Metastasectomy

All patients should be discussed at an MDT and a consensus opinion reached. Patients should be involved in the process and fully understanding of any risk/benefit associated with any individual case. All patients identified with an adrenal lesion suspected of being a metastasis and considered for surgical resection should undergo:

- Biochemical screening to exclude pheochromocytoma and hypercortisolemia.
- CXR.
- PET scanning to establish the presence or absence of further metastases.
- CT/MRI of abdomen and chest.
- Octreotide/MIBI scanning if a neuroendocrine tumor (NET) is the primary.
- Biopsy should only be considered when imaging is equivocal.

Known Disseminated Metastatic Disease Present

- Consider alternative forms of palliation alternative, e.g., radiotherapy/radiofrequency ablation.
- In the presence of widespread metastatic disease, metastasectomy should only be considered where lesions are highly symptomatic (painful), and alternative palliation is either not effective or not suitable.
- If patient life expectancy is short, then palliative analgesic treatment is advised.
- In some rare cases, when widespread metastases are known but life expectancy may be extended (e.g., NET), symptomatic adrenal metastases may be resected.

Isolated Synchronous Adrenal Metastasis

- Diagnosed usually on PET/CT at initial presentation of the primary tumor, these lesions are almost certainly indicative of widespread disease.
- Leave 3/6 months and reevaluate.
- After 6 months if still isolated single lesion, consider removal.
- Exception to this is ipsilateral adrenal metastasis with renal cell cancer as a radial nephrectomy includes adrenalectomy.

Isolated Metachronous Adrenal Metastases

- Diagnosed on follow-up >6 months after primary treatment
- PET/octreotide scan to establish whether evidence of other occult diseases (if positive then as above)
- Renal cell cancers often not PET positive
- Surgical removal of true isolated adrenal metastases:

  - Laparoscopic adrenalectomy preferred surgical option
  - Open adrenalectomy when appropriate (local invasion)

Removal of a second isolated metastasis in the remaining adrenal gland will render the patient permanently steroid dependant. This clinical situation is very rare without evidence of other metastatic disease and should only be considered in exceptional circumstances. The likely primary to cause this situation is renal cell cancer.

In all patients surgery should be performed with minimal morbidity and be considered only when quality of life will be significantly enhanced.

Pearls and Pitfalls

Pearls	Pitfalls
All patients should be discussed in a multidisciplinary team (MDT) meeting	Be sure that the imaging is contemporaneous as some adrenal metastases have a rapid doubling time (esp melanoma)
Distinguish between synchronous and metachronous disease	"Symptomatic" metastases are more likely to be associated with local invasion
Be prepared to undertake extensive laparoscopic adhesiolysis if the primary tumor was intraperitoneal	Resist becoming the "technician" for unfamiliar cancer MDTs to your practice – always discuss cases with the relevant oncologist

Further Reading

Kim SH, Brennan MF, Russo P, Burt ME, Coit DG. The role of surgery in the treatment of clinically isolated adrenal metastases. Cancer. 1998;82(2):389–94.

Mueller-Lisse UG, Mueller-Lisse UL. Imaging of advanced renal cell carcinoma. World J Urol. 2010;28(3):253–61.

Sancho JJ, Triponez F, Montet X, Sitges-Serra A. Surgical management of adrenal metastases. Langenbecks Arch Surg. 2012;397(2):179–94.

Chapter 7
Minimally Invasive Adrenal Surgery

Barney Harrison

Let us assume that the indications for surgery are correct and the patient is appropriately prepared and consented for operation (including the need for conversion to open surgery if need be). This is not a description of how to perform adrenalectomy but tips and tricks and cautions.

General Advice

Do not grab adrenal tissue with any instrument – it will fracture and bleed.
   Remember conversion to open surgery is not a "failure"; patient safety is all.
   Avoid dividing vessels close to the tumor capsule:

- Heat from the vessel sealing instrument can lead to capsule rupture.
- Subsequent pressure from "retraction" will cause them to bleed.

Transperitoneal Adrenalectomy

Use 10+ mm ports to allow complete flexibility and exchange of instruments.
   It helps if you are able to use right and left hands for any role.
   Be flexible in terms of which port gives you the best view with the camera.

B. Harrison, MBBS, MS, FRCS Eng
Department of Endocrine Surgery,
Royal Hallamshire Hospital, Glossop Road,
Sheffield S10 2JF, UK
e-mail: barney.harrison@sth.nhs.uk, barneyharrison@btinternet.com

J.C. Watkinson, D.M. Scott-Coombes (eds.), *Tips and Tricks in Endocrine Surgery*,
DOI 10.1007/978-1-4471-2146-6_7, © Springer-Verlag London 2014

Position

Almost lateral position for transperitoneal adrenalectomy with the operating table break opened at the waist of the patient. Do not overdo it as this may cause narrowing of the inferior vena cava (IVC) and hypotension due to impaired venous return. Place the operating table in a slight head up position; this allows the viscera to fall inferiorly away from the operative field. Bring the patient as close as possible to the edge of the table on the surgeon's side.

Mark the costal margin prior to insufflation as sometimes it is difficult to palpate when the abdomen is full of CO_2. The ports should not be too close to the costal margin as this may make closure of the rectus sheath difficult at the end of the procedure. In case of conversion if the port sites are at least one finger breadth from the costal margin, they can be included in the subcostal wound.

Right Adrenalectomy

Use an open method to achieve insertion of the first port in order to minimize the risk of liver injury. Four ports are required.

The key to the initial part of the operation is upward traction on the liver to divide the peritoneum between the liver and adrenal/tumor. The primary surgeon is the best judge of the required tension necessary for this retraction.

On first elevation of the anterior border of the liver, check there are no adhesions between its undersurface and the peritoneum overlying the superficial aspect of the kidney or adrenal. If the liver capsule tears, this causes blood to drip into the operative field and is a potential site of worsening liver injury due to liver retraction.

Divide the right triangular ligament of the liver as much as you can to facilitate opening the gap between the adrenal and the lower border of the liver in front of the posterior abdominal wall. Divide the peritoneum at the inferior border of the liver as far as the lateral border of the IVC.

Find the anterior aspect of the kidney near to the upper pole and dissect onto the renal capsule. Extend the dissection through the perirenal fat laterally and posteriorly onto the posterior abdominal wall. Divide the peritoneum on the lateral aspect of the adrenal but not completely; otherwise, the tumor will "fall" towards the IVC. Mobilize on the posterior aspect of the adrenal and tumor in the plane just superficial to the muscle of the abdominal wall. This facilitates later lateral retraction of the tumor from the IVC.

Watch out for vessels at three sites:

(a) Just below the inferior border of the liver on the posterior abdominal wall
(b) Running from the renal pedicle to the adrenal just lateral to the IVC
(c) Posteriorly at the lateral border of the IVC

When the adrenal/tumor is mobilized on its superior, lateral, and inferior aspects, the caval side remains. Safe and appropriate use of whichever vessel sealing instrument you use is important to avoid incomplete division of the vessels in the plane posterior to the IVC that run transversely to and from the tumor – if they bleed it can be troublesome to stop them. There may be small accessory adrenal veins entering the IVC – treat them with respect. Be gentle with the adrenal vein!

Left Side

Three ports will usually suffice.

Divide any congenital adhesions just above the splenic flexure that will impair access of the camera or instruments via the most lateral port.

Mobilization of the splenic flexure of the colon is rarely required.

Gentle retraction on the lateral border of the spleen allows clear visualization of the peritoneum on its lateral border. This should be divided approximately 1 cm from the edge of the spleen inferiorly as far as its lower border and superiorly to have clear view of the greater curve/fundus of the stomach. It is better to initially only divide the peritoneum rather than the deeper layers during this maneuver to ensure there is no irritating bleeding from the deeper fatty tissue that will hamper your view.

Full mobilization of the spleen allows for access onto the posterior abdominal wall between the posterior border of the reflected pancreatic tail and the medial border of the adrenal/tumor.

Superiorly, division of fatty tissue starts the dissection of this "gutter" which is crucial to access and mobilize the medial border of the adrenal/tumor. A phrenic vein will usually be apparent as the dissection progresses in an inferior direction and can be divided. The difficult area for this medial mobilization is the lower part of the gutter, as the access to the inferomedial aspect of the adrenal/tumor is often limited by the pancreas which may tend to fall into the operative view. To combat this:

- Check that the spleen (and pancreas) has been fully mobilized.
- Facilitate lateral retraction of the adrenal/tumor.
  Start dissecting through the fat on the upper pole of the kidney, identify the renal capsule, and then dissect immediately medial to the medial border of the kidney onto the posterior abdominal wall – superiorly towards the diaphragm and inferiorly to just above the renal pedicle. Mobilize the posterior border of the adrenal/tumor (from medial and lateral aspects) in the plane just superficial to the muscles of the posterior abdominal wall.

From the inferomedial corner the inferior dissection continues laterally with the aim of identifying and dividing the adrenal vein. Thinning the tissue from the anterior aspect of the adrenal just above the renal pedicle from the lateral and/or medial direction allows for upward retraction of the gland with a pledgelet which helps to display the vessels.

In obese patients it may be helpful at this point to insert a 4th port (5 mm) to allow inferior retraction of the fatty tissue just above the lateral transverse colon in order to better access the upper border of the renal pedicle/inferior border of the adrenal.

General Tips

Do not divide the superior attachments of the gland/tumor until all else is free; otherwise, it will fall inferiorly onto the renovascular pedicle.

Adverse anatomy will sometimes place the tail of the pancreas at risk just posterior and lateral or inferior to the spleen. Remember the pancreas is pink and the adrenal yellow and the risk is greater in obese patients when the view is poor. The tail of the pancreas will be more anterior than an adrenal gland; if in doubt dissect just lateral to the structure – if it is the pancreas, it will have fat posterior to it and move with medial retraction of the spleen.

Watch out for vessels in addition to phrenic and adrenal veins such as an adrenal artery arising from the distal renal artery and occasional upper pole vessels to the kidney.

Do not forget to unbreak the table prior to tumor extraction from the abdomen.

- This allows for easier removal of the specimen and through the smallest incision.
- Closure of the wounds is free of tension.

In patients with ACTH-dependant Cushing's or when an adrenal lesion is small in the presence of excess retroperitoneal fat:

- Do not worry if you cannot see the adrenal. You should aim to remove the adrenal gland within the fat according to the method above – the gland will be there!
- Avoid dissecting close to the adrenal capsule. If the gland is incompletely removed, the hormonal syndrome will persist/recur because of the high levels of ACTH.

If intraoperative injury to the diaphragm occurs, usually during right adrenalectomy at division of the right triangular ligament of the liver, you may see a hole or notice that the hemidiaphragm has become very floppy. Inform the anesthetist and continue the procedure. At the end of the operation, ask the anesthetist to inflate the lungs manually, release the pneumoperitoneum, and remove the ports. Ask for a chest X-ray in recovery. A small pneumothorax in the absence of any other confounding morbidity requires no intervention.

Posterior Retroperitoneoscopic Adrenalectomy (PRPA)

A team effort is required because key issues are applying the anesthetic and correct positioning of the patient. If you are planning to start to use this approach, take members of the theater team to an appropriate center where you and they can see what is required in terms of the positioning, instrumentation, and operative technique.

Advantages of PRPA: A very good view and lack of need to mobilize liver, spleen, and pancreas; on the right side, the vessels posterior to the IVC and the adrenal vein/s are much easier to control. The higher gas pressure used in retroperitoneal surgery (at least 20 mmHg) reduces bleeding to a minimum. Bilateral adrenalectomy can be performed without need for repositioning.

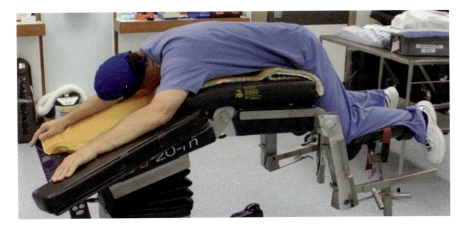

Fig. 7.1 Patient position for posterior retroperitoneoscopic adrenalectomy

Disadvantages of PRPA: The lack of familiar anatomical landmarks, a small working space, a steep learning curve, and a requirement to be able to use either hand for dissection/use of the VSI.

Indications: Smaller tumors (<5 cm)/previous major upper abdominal surgery and or upper intra-abdominal post-sepsis/hepatosplenomegaly/reoperative adrenalectomy.

General Tips

When you perform this the first few times, find a friendly mentor to come and support you. Chose the "correct" patient with the "correct" adrenal tumor.

Do not attempt to perform PRPA if the patient has undergone ipsilateral nephrectomy.

It may be difficult to find the plane between the kidney and perirenal fat in the patient with prior recurrent upper urinary tract infection.

PRPA for tumors at the lower pole of the adrenal abutting the renal pedicle is more difficult.

Positioning

See Fig. 7.1

The patient is positioned prone with hips and knees flexed, with the side of surgery as near to the side of the operating table as can be achieved. Try to minimize the lumbar lordosis with the aid of a small amount of table break and/or an oval or rectangular support under the patients abdomen that allows the abdomen to fall freely onto the surface of the operating table (not essential but may help in obese patients).

Ensure that there is sufficient padding under the patient at the hips, upper thighs, and weight-bearing surface of the tibiae. The arms are placed on boards with the hands pointing towards the anesthetist; the face should be suitably protected from pressure damage.

Pearls

When the patient is correctly positioned, mark the tip of the 12th rib before you scrub – it may be more difficult to palpate with your gloves on.

Make a transverse incision onto the tip of the 12th rib, and from this point try to avoid stretching this incision any more than you need as a gas leak through the muscle incision makes the procedure much more tedious and increases the chance and extent of surgical emphysema. Just below the tip of the rib, push the scissors through the muscle (guarding against too deep penetration) – you will feel a "pop" as you do it. Spread the jaws at the muscle layer to enlarge this hole to a size to admit your index finger.

Sweep the fat and fascia off the anterior aspect of the muscle; medially your finger will palpate the paraspinal muscles, laterally the tip of the 11th rib. Insert the medial port (10 mm) obliquely, the lateral port (5 mm), and then the blocking port. On insertion of the medial and lateral ports, you must guard the port tip with your finger as it comes through the body wall.

Insufflate and insert the telescope (30°) turned to look upwards via the middle port.

"Find" the tips of the grasping forceps inserted via the other ports and then identify Gerota's fascia. Open the fascia – if you do this slightly too far laterally, you will open the peritoneum in error; it does not matter:

- Divide all the "filmy" adhesions on the posterior aspect of the upper half of the kidney.
- Create the working space using the paraspinal muscles to orientate yourself.
- Dissect through perirenal fat onto the renal capsule at the upper pole of the kidney.
- Clear the fat from the upper pole deep to the fat, on the capsule, so the kidney is freely mobile on all aspects – this is really important!
- If mobilized perirenal fat gets in the way – excise it and push it out of the way.

As the kidney becomes more mobile, you will need to rotate the port to look "down" and be flexible in using the medial or middle ports to obtain the best view.

You can now start to mobilize the adrenal/tumor on its lateral, anterior, and medial borders. Leave the superior attachments of the adrenal until the very end.

If the kidney upper pole is sufficiently mobile, access to the inferior pole of the adrenal is markedly easier.

At right adrenalectomy, be careful as you mobilize the anterior aspect of the adrenal that you do not go too far medially; the lateral border of the IVC is at risk.

For this reason, the IVC should be delineated and the medial aspect of the adrenal/tumor cleared from its posterior aspect.

At the end of the procedure, reduce the CO_2 pressure sufficient to maintain the space and confirm hemostasis.

If the anesthetist reports that the end tidal (or arterial) CO_2 is too high, stop and release the pneumoretroperitoneum until you are informed that you can start again.

Surgical emphysema is very common because of the high insufflation pressures and long operation. Reassure everyone who is worried that it will settle.

Postoperatively

Patients in the first 24/48 h after PRPA have less pain and are more mobile.

A recognized complication of PRPA is subcostal nerve injury, nearly always temporary, caused at port insertion. It may be evident in the recovery ward as abdominal swelling and concern expressed by the nursing staff or, subsequently, by the patient. Reassurance is usually all that is required.

Further Reading

Alesina PF, Hommeltenberg S, Meier B, Petersenn S, Lahner H, Schmid KW, et al. Posterior retroperitoneoscopic adrenalectomy for clinical and subclinical Cushing's syndrome. World J Surg. 2010;34(6):1391–7.

Dickson PV, Jimenez C, Chisholm GB, Kennamer DL, Ng C, Grubbs EG, et al. Posterior retroperitoneoscopic adrenalectomy: a contemporary American experience. J Am Coll Surg. 2011;212(4):659–65; discussion 665–7.

Part II
Pancreas/Neuroendocrine

Chapter 8
Diagnosis and Preoperative Assessment (Algorithms) for Pancreatic NETs

Rachel Troke and Karim Meeran

Definition of Pancreatic Neuroendocrine Tumors (pNETs) and Subdivisions

PNETs arise from neuroendocrine cells within the pancreas. Most (up to 90 % in some series) do not secrete hormones (nonfunctioning) and may be an incidental finding on imaging. The rest are described as functioning. These exhibit hypersecretion of various hormones and are generally defined by their secretory products. They may produce one or more hormones, which subsequently give rise to a specific clinical picture (Table 8.1).

Epidemiology and Pathology

PNETs are rare, occurring with an incidence of less than 1:100,000. However, postmortem findings suggest that these tumors are more common than previously thought, up to 10 % in some studies. Many small tumors that are nonfunctioning, and therefore asymptomatic, remain undiagnosed. Patients with functioning tumors are more likely to be symptomatic and so tend to be diagnosed at a younger age. Overall survival is better in those with functional lesions although it is important to bear in mind that lesions found incidentally on screening may otherwise have been one of those that patients would otherwise have never known about. Aggressive treatment of such lesions may suggest that whatever treatment is used is effective, leading to publication bias in favor of surgical or other treatment.

R. Troke (✉) • K. Meeran
Department of Endocrinology, Imperial Centre for Endocrinology,
Hammersmith Hospital Campus,
Du Cane Road, London W12 0HS, UK
e-mail: k.meeran@imperial.ac.uk

J.C. Watkinson, D.M. Scott-Coombes (eds.), *Tips and Tricks in Endocrine Surgery*,
DOI 10.1007/978-1-4471-2146-6_8, © Springer-Verlag London 2014

Table 8.1 Clinical features associated with different types of pancreatic NET

Tumor Type	Symptoms
Insulinoma	Hypoglycemic episodes
	Sweating, tremulousness, tachycardia, hunger
	Neuroglycopenic symptoms
	Headache, lethargy, diplopia
	Seizures, loss of consciousness
	Weight gain
Gastrinoma	Zollinger-Ellison syndrome
	Abdominal pain from multiple gastroduodenal ulcers
	Upper GI bleed or perforation
	Heartburn or acid reflux
	Diarrhea
	Nausea and vomiting
	Weight loss
	Symptoms may respond to high-dose PPI
VIPoma	Profound watery secretory diarrhea
	Electrolyte disturbance (hypokalemia)
	Lethargy
	Nausea and vomiting
	Abdominal pain
Glucagonoma	Hyperglucagonemia, hyperglycemia
	Weight loss
	Diarrhea
	Stomatitis
	Necrolytic migratory erythema
	Erythematous blistering rash seen over lower abdomen, perineum, and groin
	Deep vein thrombosis
Somatostatinoma	Diabetes/impaired glucose tolerance
	Gallstones/gallbladder disease
	Diarrhea/steatorrhea
	Weight loss
	Abdominal pain
Nonfunctioning	No hormonal hypersecretion
	Late presentation therefore often metastatic
	Nonspecific abdominal symptoms often due to tumor mass or local invasion
	Abdominal pain
	Weight loss, anorexia, nausea
	Jaundice

Nonfunctioning pNETS are classified using the WHO scheme, ranging from well-differentiated endocrine carcinomas with a Ki67 index of <2 % to poorly differentiated lesions with high-grade malignant behavior and a Ki67 index usually >20 %. The majority of nonfunctioning pNETs fall into the former category.

Genetic Associations

Most cases of pNETs occur sporadically, but there are some associations with genetic syndromes such as multiple endocrine neoplasia type 1 (MEN-1), tuberous sclerosis, and von Hippel-Lindau disease (VHL). In VHL and tuberous sclerosis, these lesions are an unusual finding and tend to be nonfunctioning.

- 25–30 % of those with gastrinoma will have underlying MEN-1, but only about 5 % of those with insulinoma will have this genetic condition.
- Careful history and examination is essential to look for other manifestations of complex genetic causes for pNET (e.g., symptoms of hypercalcemia, renal stones, or symptoms of pituitary lesions in MEN-1).
- Genetic testing should be carried out in all young patients presenting with pNET.
- A careful family history for potential unrecognized manifestations of a genetic condition should be taken.

Investigations

Patients should be investigated in a systematic manner (Fig. 8.1).

Biochemical

The use of biochemical markers in pNETs is useful for both diagnosis and also in the long-term follow-up of patients after surgical or medical therapy. Some assays are commercially available, but it is often necessary to send specific samples to regional centers such as the Hammersmith Hospital (London, UK). Always liaise with your local laboratory to inform them you will be sending them samples for gut hormones to avoid delays in processing and subsequent degradation of hormone within the sample.

- *Chromogranin A and B* are nonspecific markers for neuroendocrine tumors and may be elevated in both functioning and nonfunctioning pNETs. Sample should be taken in two EDTA tubes, sent immediately to the lab on ice, and spun straight away.
- *Pancreatic polypeptide* (PP) is a general marker which is seen to be elevated in 50–80 % of pNETs. It should be collected in the same manner as chromogranin A and B.
- *Insulin* can be measured in suspected insulinoma, but should be taken only when the patient is hypoglycemic (<2.2 mmol/L). Hypoglycemia may be spontaneous or achieved within the context of a 72-h supervised fast. A plain clotted tube should be sent for insulin and C-peptide measurement, with a matched sample for glucose. In insulinoma, the insulin level will be inappropriately raised in the context of hypoglycemia. (A lack of concurrent rise of C-peptide suggests exogenous insulin

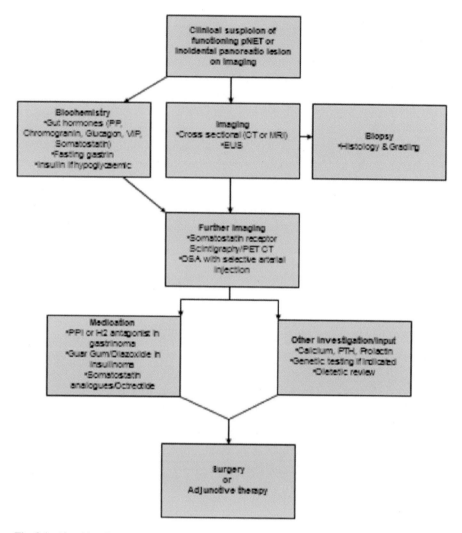

Fig. 8.1 Algorithm for preoperative management of pancreatic NETs

administration. A sulfonylurea screen should also be sent in a plain clotted tube, as sulfonylureas will give a raised insulin and C-peptide with hypoglycemia.)

- *Gastrin* is elevated in gastrinomas, although some pNETs may secrete more than one hormonal product. It should be measured in the fasting state. In gastrinomas, levels >40 pmol/L will be seen. Gastrin can be artificially elevated by proton pump inhibitors (PPIs), H2 antagonists, pernicious anemia, other causes of achlorhydria, and renal failure. Ideally PPIs should be stopped 2 weeks prior to gastrin measurement and substituted with an H2 blocker which is then stopped 48–72 h prior to blood sampling for gastrin. (In some patients with gastrinoma, it may be impossible or even dangerous to stop PPI therapy.) Samples should be taken in 2 EDTA tubes, stored on ice, and spun and separated within 15 min.

In some cases of suspected gastrinoma where fasting gastrin results have been equivocal, it may be helpful to consider an intravenous secretin test. In gastrinoma, gastrin levels rise after IV secretin, while in normal individuals, gastrin levels should fall. Ideally both PPI and H2 antagonists should be stopped prior to the procedure, but the test will still provide useful diagnostic information if the patient is unable to stop these medications.

- *Glucagon, vasoactive intestinal peptide (VIP), and somatostatin* should also be collected in 2 EDTA tubes and separated immediately. These can be measured in suspected glucagonomas, VIPomas, and somatostatinomas, respectively.
- *Calcium, parathyroid hormone, and prolactin* should be measured in any patient with a pNET, particularly gastrinoma, due to the association with MEN1 syndrome.

Imaging

See Chap. 9

Preoperative Management

General

- Always refer to a multidisciplinary team in a referral center for pNETs.
- Surgery should be performed in a specialist hepatobiliary unit by a surgeon with extensive experience in management of pNETs.

Insulinoma

- Involve the dietician for advice on small, regular meals.
- Consider guar gum 5 g tds or diazoxide 50–200 mg tds.
- NG feeding may be required if symptoms are severe.
- Octreotide s/c can be useful.

Gastrinoma

- Continue PPI and/or H2 antagonist to control symptoms and reduce the risk of upper GI bleeding.
- If patients are unable to stop PPI/H2 antagonist for investigations, consider a secretin test.

Inoperable Lesions

- Surgical debulking may help in symptom control.
- Ablative therapy with chemoembolization, selective internal radiation therapy (SIRT), or radiofrequency ablation is usually used for palliation of hepatic metastases, often to ameliorate symptoms of hormonal overactivity.
- Systemic or adjuvant chemotherapy may be useful in some patients.
- Peptide receptor radionuclide therapy (PRRT) is a relatively novel treatment that couples a somatostatin analogue with radionuclides such as ^{90}Yttrium or ^{177}Lutetium. These radionuclides target lesions that are proven to have high avidity on somatostatin receptor scintigraphy (i.e., lots of somatostatin receptors) and have shown some success in tumor shrinkage.

Pearls and Pitfalls

Pearls	Pitfalls
Patients should be managed in experienced centers	Beware exogenous hyperinsulinemia (measure C-peptide)
Work in a multidisciplinary team	Avoid the temptation to rush to surgery – invest time in stabilizing the effects of excess hormone secretion and preoperative nutrition
Biochemical tests should precede imaging	Do not miss MEN-1

Further Reading

Dhillo WS, Jayasena CN, Jackson JE, Lynn JA, Bloom SR, Meeran K, et al. Localization of gastrinomas by selective intra-arterial calcium injection in patients on proton pump inhibitor or H2 receptor antagonist therapy. Eur J Gastroenterol Hepatol. 2005;17(4):429–33.

Fein J, Gerdes H. Localization of islet cell tumors by endoscopic ultrasonography. Gastroenterology. 1992;103(2):711–2.

Halfdanarson TR, Rabe KG, Rubin J, Petersen GM. Pancreatic neuroendocrine tumours (PNETs): incidence, prognosis and recent trend towards improved survival. Ann Oncol. 2008;19:1727–33.

Imperial Centre for Endocrinology. http://impce.com.

European Neuroendocrine Tumor Society. http://www.enets.org/guidelines.

National Cancer Institute. Surveillance, epidemiology, and end results (SEER) Stat Fact Sheets. 2013. http://seer.cancer.gov.

Ramage JK, Ahmed A, Ardill J, Bax N, Breen DJ, Caplin ME, et al. Guidelines for the management of gastroenteropancreatic neuroendocrine (including carcinoid) tumours (NETs). Gut. 2012;61(1):6–32. Epub 2011 Nov 3.

Turner JJ, Wren AM, Jackson JE, Thakker RV, Meeran K. Localization of gastrinomas by selective intra-arterial calcium injection. Clin Endocrinol. 2002;57(6):821–5.

Chapter 9
Localization of Pancreatic and Gastrointestinal NETs

James E. Jackson and Tara D. Barwick

Introduction

- The imaging of gastroenteropancreatic (GEP) neuroendocrine tumors is best discussed by dividing them into two groups:

    - Functioning insulinomas and gastrinomas. Owing to the potency of the hormone that they produce, they are almost invariably small at presentation and imaging is usually aimed at localization of the primary tumor (and exclusion of metastatic disease) with a view to surgical excision if possible.
    - Nonfunctioning or those that secrete a variety of less potent hormones (glucagon, vasoactive intestinal polypeptide, 5-hydroxytryptamine, somatostatin, serotonin, and pancreatic polypeptide). By the time that patients develop symptoms, the primary tumors are usually large and may indeed have already metastasized. The role of imaging in this group is usually that of documenting the extent of disease to guide operative or nonoperative therapy.

Functioning Insulinomas

Incidence

Insulinomas are rare and small (<1 cm) (see Chap. 10).

- The so-called adult idiopathic nesidioblastosis is an extremely rare condition in which there is diffuse β-cell hyperplasia and resultant hyperinsulinemic

J.E. Jackson, FRCP, FRCR (✉)
Department of Imaging, Hammersmith Hospital, Du Cane Road, London W12 0HS, UK
e-mail: jejacks@googlemail.com

T.D. Barwick, MSc, MRCP, FRCR
Department of Imaging, Imperial College Healthcare NHS Trust,
Hammersmith Hospital, Du Cane Road, London W12 0HS, UK
e-mail: tara.barwick@imperial.nhs.uk

J.C. Watkinson, D.M. Scott-Coombes (eds.), *Tips and Tricks in Endocrine Surgery*,
DOI 10.1007/978-1-4471-2146-6_9, © Springer-Verlag London 2014

hypoglycemia. None of the various imaging modalities discussed below will allow a preoperative diagnosis, which can only be made by biopsy.

Imaging of Insulinomas

- No patient should undergo imaging until a biochemical diagnosis of hyperinsulinemic hypoglycemia has been confirmed.
- While an experienced surgeon using direct palpation of the pancreas together with intraoperative ultrasound scanning will be able to localize an insulinoma in close to 100 % of cases, most surgeons agree that preoperative localization is helpful in that it usually reduces the duration of surgery and may limit the extent of pancreatic resection.
- Precise tumor localization is essential when a laparoscopy is to be used as patient positioning on the operating table and the surgical approach will vary depending upon the site of the neoplasm.

Computed Tomography

- Arguably the most useful noninvasive investigation is contrast-enhanced multidetector computed tomography (MDCT). Best results are obtained with a technique that includes oral water loading, bowel paralysis, and data acquisition during both arterial and portal venous phases of contrast medium enhancement. The typical findings are of a well-defined nodule within the pancreas that enhances avidly during the arterial phase study (Fig. 9.1).
- With a biochemical diagnosis of an insulinoma in whom the CT shows the typical appearances of a single intrapancreatic neuroendocrine tumor, there is a good argument for referring the patient for surgical resection at this stage without further imaging although endoscopic ultrasound may still provide important additional information such as the relationship of the tumor to the pancreatic duct.
- Despite recent advances in MDCT, there will still be a significant number of patients in whom a tumor will not be visualized, and these individuals will need further investigation.

Endoscopic Ultrasound (EUS)

- In experienced hands, this investigation is recognized as being one of the most sensitive modalities for the detection of small intrapancreatic neoplasms with detection rates in several series of over 90 %.
- The entire pancreas can be examined in the majority of individuals; the body and tail of the pancreas are imaged through the gastric wall and the pancreatic head via the duodenum. High-frequency transducers (8–12 MHz) are used, and tumors as small as 5 mm may be detected.

Fig. 9.1 (**a**) Axial CT image during the arterial phase of contrast medium enhancement demonstrates a brightly enhancing 8 mm diameter nodule (*arrow*) in the anterior portion of the pancreatic head consistent with an insulinoma. (**b**) Axial CT image in the same patient demonstrates a second brightly enhancing 3 mm diameter nodule (*arrow*) in the pancreatic tail. (**c**) Single image from coeliac axis arteriogram demonstrates both tumor nodules (*arrows*). Arterial stimulation venous sampling performed during the same procedure confirmed that the pancreatic head lesion secreted insulin and that the tail lesion was nonfunctioning. The patient went on to have a curative laparoscopic enucleation of the pancreatic head tumor

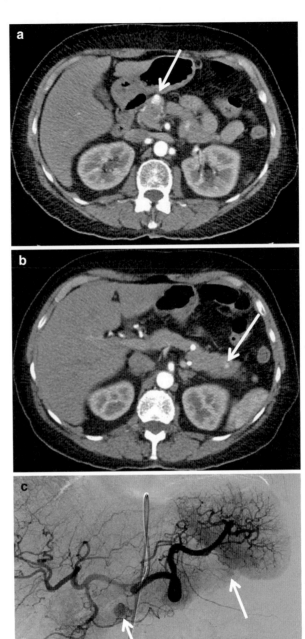

- Most tumors will be markedly hypervascular on color Doppler ultrasound, and tumor conspicuity may be further enhanced by using intravenous "bubble" contrast medium.
- Fine-needle aspiration cytology can also be performed although this is rarely necessary if a single neoplasm is seen in the context of hyperinsulinemic hypoglycemia.

Magnetic Resonance (MR) Imaging

- As with CT, a meticulous scanning technique, including bowel paralysis, is important, and intravenous enhancement with gadolinium may be required. Tumors are usually of low signal intensity on T1-weighted images, especially if fat suppression sequences are used, and will show enhancement following intravenous contrast medium. On T2-weighted images, tumors are more likely to be hyper- or isointense when compared with the normal surrounding pancreatic parenchyma.
- The reported sensitivity for the detection of primary pancreatic insulinomas varies considerably from as low as 20 % to one approaching 100 %; a figure of between 50 and 70 % is probably reasonable.
- MR will not infrequently demonstrate tumors which have not been localized on MDCT particularly in patients with MEN1. Those patients in whom there is biochemical evidence of a functioning insulinoma, but have multiple pancreatic neoplasms, will usually require further investigation (often angiography combined with arterial stimulation venous sampling) if surgical excision is being considered to try and determine which of the tumors is functioning.

Radionuclide Imaging

Radiolabeled Somatostatin Analogs

- A variety of tumors, both neuroendocrine and non-neuroendocrine, contain somatostatin receptors (SSTr). NETs frequently express a high density of SSTr, particularly the SSTr2 subtype, which forms the molecular basis for somatostatin receptor scintigraphy. Somatostatin receptor scintigraphy (SRS) with [111] Indium-DTPA-octreotide (^{111}In-octreotide) has proved to be highly sensitive in localizing and documenting the extent of disease in the majority of these neoplasms with reported sensitivities of 75–100 %. The one exception is insulinomas for which the reported sensitivities are 40–60 % due to their lower incidence of somatostatin receptors in general and of the subtype 2 in particular.

Positron Emission Tomography (PET) Combined with CT (PET-CT)

- PET using 18-fluorodeoxyglucose (FDG), a glucose analog, has become very useful in general oncology but has a limited role in the investigation of pancreatic neuroendocrine tumors and, in particular, insulinomas due to the relatively slow metabolic rate of NET cells.

Fig. 9.2 (**a**) Axial CT image during the arterial phase of contrast medium enhancement demonstrates a 12 mm diameter brightly enhancing tumor in the pancreatic body (*arrow*) consistent with an insulinoma. (**b**) Single fused image from [68]Gallium DOTATATE PET-CT study demonstrates intense uptake of the radionuclide within the tumor. No other abnormal uptake was seen. The patient went on to have curative laparoscopic resection

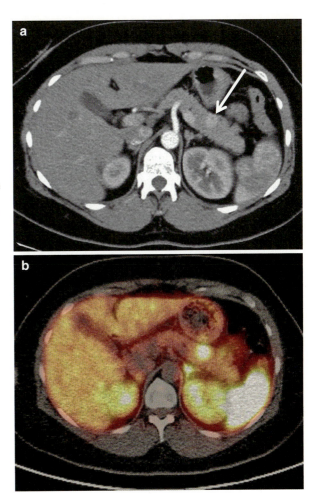

- More recently, [68]Gallium-DOTA peptide PET imaging has shown greater promise in the documentation of disease extent for both low- and high-grade GEP tumors, and there is recent evidence that it, and other newer PET isotopes, may help localize small insulinomas (Fig. 9.2).
- In general, [68]Gallium-DOTA peptide PET imaging has superseded SRS with ^{111}In-octreotide due to its higher binding affinity and different receptor profile with resultant greater accumulation of radiotracer in SSTr positive cells. Furthermore, the higher spatial resolution of PET images when compared with those obtained by SPECT permits the detection of smaller lesions. There are other advantages:

  - The study is completed in 2 h while ^{111}In-octreotide imaging requires longer acquisition times and is performed over 2 days.
  - The tracer is cheaper as it is generator produced.

Unfortunately, however, [68]Gallium-DOTA peptide PET imaging is currently not widely available largely due to regulatory issues regarding manufacturing authorization; this should be overcome in the near future.

Angiography and Arterial Stimulation Venous Sampling

- Visceral angiography with arterial stimulation venous sampling (ASVS) used to be considered the most sensitive investigation for the detection of insulinomas but is now less frequently necessary. The indications for its use are:
  - When the other investigations described above have failed to identify an intrapancreatic neoplasm
  - When there is more than one intrapancreatic neoplasm and information is required about function to direct localized surgical resection (Fig. 9.1c)
- Localization of an insulinoma by ASVS relies upon a detectable rise in insulin in hepatic venous samples after the selective injection of calcium gluconate in turn into the arteries supplying different portions of the pancreas. It only localizes the tumor to a region of the pancreas rather than to a specific site if the angiogram does not demonstrate a tumor blush. It has the advantage, however, of being able to confirm that a visualized angiographic abnormality is a functioning tumor.

Functioning Gastrinomas

- Sixty percent of gastrinomas are multicentric or have metastasized at the time of diagnosis and 40 % are extrapancreatic, most commonly within the duodenum.
- Like insulinomas, the primary tumors and lymph node metastases are usually small (less than 1 cm in diameter) at the time of diagnosis due to the potent effect of gastrin.
- Approximately 30 % of patients with a gastrinoma will have multiple endocrine neoplasia type 1 (MEN1) and such individuals are more likely to have multiple duodenal tumors.
- The vast majority (approximately 90 %) of these neoplasms occur within the "gastrinoma triangle," an area bounded by the junction of the neck and body of the pancreas medially, the junction of the second and third parts of the duodenum inferiorly, and the junction of the cystic and common bile ducts superiorly.
- Tumors within the duodenum are often less than 5 mm in diameter and are notoriously difficult to localize preoperatively.

Imaging of Gastrinomas

Much of the information regarding the imaging of insulinomas also applies to gastrinomas, but there are some important differences, which will be discussed below.

Radionuclide Imaging

Radiolabeled Somatostatin Analogs

- Unlike insulinomas the majority of gastrinomas contain a high density of somatostatin receptors, and this form of imaging is extremely useful for the localization of primary tumors and for the demonstration of distant spread to regional
  lymph nodes or the liver.
- There is a good argument in favor of performing this investigation first and only proceed-
  ing to other imaging studies if the SRS is negative and surgery is being contemplated.
- The combination of single-photon emission computed tomography (SPECT)
  images fused with low-dose computed tomography improves the sensitivity of
  the investigation.
- SRS is one of the most sensitive preoperative imaging studies for extrahepatic
  gastrinomas but may still miss one-third of all lesions found at surgery. Negative
  results of SRS should not, therefore, be used to decide operability.
- SRS has an important role in surgical follow-up and in evaluating the response to
  other therapies.

Positron Emission Tomography (PET) Combined with CT (PET-CT)

- Most gastrinomas have a low proliferation rate, and FDG-PET is generally
  unhelpful. Those tumors with an aggressive clinical behavior are usually less
  well differentiated and may as a result be negative on SRS but show intense FDG
  uptake because of a higher proliferative activity. In such cases FDG-PET is of
  prognostic significance and may alter the therapeutic approach.
- [68]Gallium-DOTA peptides have recently been shown to be of greater value than
  FDG in the documentation of disease extent in well-differentiated GEP tumors
  and may also have a role in the imaging of poorly differentiated neoplasms, as
  tumor heterogeneity in terms of receptor positivity and degree of differentiation
  may be present in different lesions in the same patient.
- These diagnostic radiopharmaceuticals also have a therapeutic application as they
  may permit selection of somatostatin receptor-positive GEP tumors which are
  inoperable and/or metastatic but suitable for targeted radionuclide therapy with
  somatostatin analogs labelled to the β-emitters [90]Yttrium or [177]Lutetium (Fig. 9.3).

Endoscopic Ultrasound

- Endoscopic ultrasound has been reported as being a highly sensitive technique
  (about 80 %) for the demonstration of both pancreatic and extrapancreatic tumors
  although small duodenal tumors may be difficult to visualize. It has been suggested

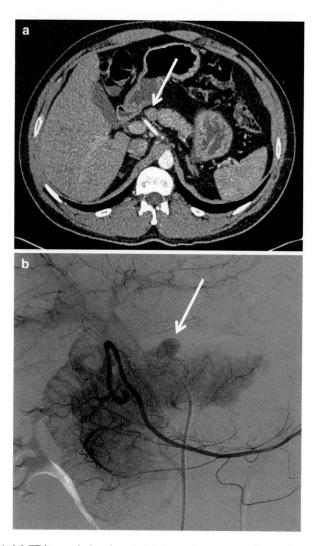

Fig. 9.3 (a) Axial CT image during the arterial phase of contrast medium enhancement demonstrates a 12 mm exopytic pancreatic neck gastrinoma (*arrow*) which enhances to a similar degree as the adjacent pancreatic parenchyma. (b) Selective gastroduodenal artery angiogram demonstrates the same exophytic pancreatic neck neoplasm (*arrow*). This tumor was successfully removed surgically. (c) Follow-up CT image obtained during the arterial phase of contrast medium enhancement demonstrates a soft tissue nodule adjacent to the anterior aspect of the low pancreatic head (*arrow*) consistent with metastatic lymphadenopathy. (d) Fused image from ^{68}Ga DOTATATE PET-CT demonstrate intense uptake of the radionuclide in the nodule confirming metastatic disease. This was the only focus of disease. The patient went on to have treatment with [177]Lutetium DOTATATE. (e) Low-dose unenhanced CT image after three [177]Lutetium DOTATATE therapy sessions documents a marked decrease in size of the metastatic lymphadenopathy (*arrow*)

Fig. 9.3 (continued)

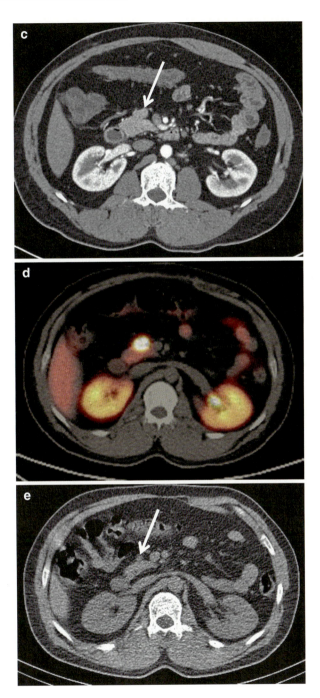

that EUS may be useful in excluding an intrapancreatic primary so that subsequent localization techniques can be aimed at finding an extrapancreatic neoplasm. Tumors may be hypo-, iso-, or hyperechoic with respect to normal pancreatic parenchyma. Contrast Doppler ultrasound may be helpful.

Computed Tomography (Fig. 9.3)

- Primary gastrinomas are usually less vascular than insulinomas, and as a result, MDCT is less good at localizing them, especially those within the duodenum. A reported sensitivity of approximately 30 % is quoted. Hepatic metastases are usually easily identified.

Visceral Angiography and Arterial Stimulation Venous Sampling

- As with insulinomas, visceral angiography is now reserved for those patients in whom other imaging investigations have failed to document a tumor or in whom multiple tumors have been documented, and information is required regarding function to direct surgery (Fig. 9.3).
- The technique of ASVS is identical to that used for insulinomas. Secretin used to be the "provocative agent" of choice, but calcium gluconate is now more commonly used as it has been shown to work just as well. When injected into the vessel supplying a gastrinoma, both of these secretagogues will produce a significant rise in gastrin concentration in the hepatic vein of at least 25 % at 20 s or 50 % at 30 s after administration; a similar rise does not occur when the injection is made into a vessel supplying normal territory.

Other Functioning and Nonfunctioning Neuroendocrine Tumors

Pancreatic Tumors

- The majority of these tumors are large at presentation, and their demonstration by transabdominal ultrasound and/or CT is rarely a problem. Their malignant potential is high, and many have metastasized at the time of diagnosis and imaging is primarily aimed at either excluding or confirming the presence of hepatic metastases or other extrapancreatic spread.
- Primary tumors are usually of inhomogeneous soft tissue density on CT and may contain areas of cystic degeneration or calcification; the latter is frequently seen in glucagonomas. They are commonly highly vascular and will, therefore, show marked contrast enhancement, which may be inhomogeneous due to areas of necrosis, on arterial phase scans.
- Most of these neoplasms express somatostatin receptors, and scintigraphy using ^{111}In-DTPA-octreotide has, until recently, been the best method for evaluating the

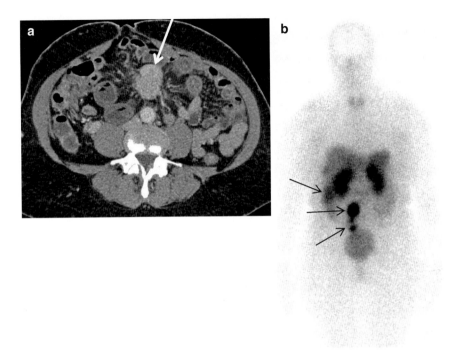

Fig. 9.4 (**a**) Axial CT image obtained during the arterial phase of contrast medium enhancement demonstrates a large enhancing mass in the small-bowel mesentery (*arrow*) consistent with metastatic lymphadenopathy from a distal ileal carcinoid tumor. Note the soft tissue stranding around this lymph node mass due to the desmoplastic reaction commonly associated with this tumor. (**b**) Whole-body planar image from ^{111}In-octreotide study demonstrates intense uptake of the radionuclide in the primary small-bowel tumor, the mesenteric lymph node mass and a metastatic deposit in the right lobe of the liver (*arrows*)

presence and extent of metastatic disease. [68]Gallium-DOTA peptide PET imaging combined with CT is now, however, considered to be the modality of choice for these tumors.

Extrapancreatic Tumors

- Midgut carcinoids are the commonest extrapancreatic neuroendocrine tumors (see Chap. 11).
- Tumors that present with small-bowel obstructive symptoms or chronic gastrointestinal blood loss may be investigated by a number of different imaging modalities, the most useful of which are:
  - CT which may show a soft tissue mass containing some calcification associated with marked stranding of the adjacent mesentery due to a surrounding desmoplastic reaction commonly associated with mesenteric venous and arterial occlusions and subsequent collaterals, small-bowel dilatation, and bowel-wall thickening (Fig. 9.4).

- The small-bowel enema (conventional barium, CT, or MR) will typically demonstrate small-bowel dilatation and angulation with thickening of the valvulae conniventes with or without an associated mass lesion.
- Angiography may demonstrate a vascular blush with associated "cork screwing," narrowing, and occlusion of the adjacent mesenteric vessels.

• In patients with carcinoid syndrome, imaging is primarily aimed at confirming the presence and extent of hepatic and extrahepatic metastases, and this is best achieved with radionuclide techniques:

- Approximately 85 % of carcinoid tumors express somatostatin receptors and scintigraphy with ^{111}In-pentetreotide as a reliable investigation for staging of disease (Fig. 9.4).
- PET-CT imaging with ^{68}Ga-DOTA peptides may also be helpful, not only to demonstrate the full extent of disease but also, in some cases, to determine whether there is any role for targeted radionuclide therapy using [90]Yttrium-DOTATOC or [177]Lutetium-DOTATATE. Both of these agents may be useful for the palliative treatment of any metastatic somatostatin receptor-positive GEP tumor.

Pearls and Pitfalls

Pearls	Pitfalls
Tailor the imaging to the NET under investigation	Lack of dedicated CT and MR imaging protocols when investigating pancreatic NETs
Ensure excellent arterial phase images during abdominal MDCT when investigating pancreatic NETs	Requirement for expert endoscopic ultrasound and visceral angiography with ASVS which are not widely available
Somatostatin receptor scintigraphy (preferably with [68]Gallium DOTA peptide PET if available) is best for delineating disease extent in metastatic gastroenteropancreatic NETs to assist selection of appropriate therapeutic approach	Underestimation of tumor load of metastatic GEP tumors by CT

Further Reading

Ambrosini V, Campana D, Tomassetti P, Fanti S. 68Ga-labelled peptides for diagnosis of gastroenteropancreatic NET. Eur J Nucl Med Mol Imaging. 2012;39 Suppl 1:S52–60.
Basu S, Kumar R, Rubello D, Fanti S, Alavi A. PET imaging in neuroendocrine tumours: current status and future prospects. Minerva Endocrinol. 2008;33:257–75.

Isla A, Arbuckle JD, Kekis PB, Lim A, Jackson JE, Todd JF, Lynn J. Laparoscopic management of insulinomas. Br J Surg. 2009;96:185–90.

Jackson JE. Angiography and arterial stimulation venous sampling in the localization of pancreatic islet cell tumours. In: Reznek RH, editor. Best practice and research. Clinical endocrinology and metabolism, vol. 19. Elsevier Science Ltd, London, UK; 2005. p. 229–39.

Kayani I, Bomanji JB, Groves A, Conway G, Gacinovic S, Win T, Dickson J, Caplin M, Ell PJ. Functional imaging of neuroendocrine tumours with combined PET/CT using 68Ga-DOTATATE (DOTA-DPhe1, Tyr3-octreotate) and 18F-FDG. Cancer. 2008;112:2447–55.

Nikfarjam M, Warshaw AL, Axelrod L, Deshpande V, Thayer SP, Ferrone CR, Fernandez-del CC. Improved contemporary surgical management of insulinomas: a 25-year experience at the Massachusetts General Hospital. Ann Surg. 2008;247:165–73.

Patel KK, Kim MK. Neuroendocrine tumors of the pancreas: endoscopic diagnosis. Curr Opin Gastroenterol. 2008;24:638–42. Review.

Rockall AG, Reznek RH. Imaging of neuroendocrine tumours (CT/MR/US). Best Pract Res Clin Endocrinol Metab. 2007;21:43–68. Review.

Chapter 10
Surgery for Pancreatic Neuroendocrine Neoplasms (pNENs)

Thomas Clerici and Bruno Schmied

pNENs

Hallmarks

- Are rare (incidence of 1/100,000; represent 1–2 % of all pancreatic neoplasms)
- Can be functional or nonfunctional in regard to hormonal hypersecretion
- Can be single or multiple
- Are often (10–20 %) associated with hereditary syndromes like multiple endocrine neoplasia type 1 (MEN1) or von Hippel-Lindau syndrome (VHL)

Presentation to the Surgeon

- Referral to surgery with a complete biochemical and imaging work-up, mostly for a specific hormonal syndrome caused by a pNEN
- Referral for the resection of a pancreatic mass of unknown origin with incomplete work-up
- As an "incidental" finding on CT or MR imaging for other pathology

T. Clerici, MD (✉) • B. Schmied, MD
Department of Surgery, Kantonsspital St. Gallen,
Rorschacherstrasse, St. Gallen CH-9007, Switzerland
e-mail: thomas.clerici@kssg.ch

J.C. Watkinson, D.M. Scott-Coombes (eds.), *Tips and Tricks in Endocrine Surgery*,
DOI 10.1007/978-1-4471-2146-6_10, © Springer-Verlag London 2014

Classification

- According to WHO 2010[1] and TNM[2] criteria

General Preoperative Considerations

- The family history regarding the possibility of multiple endocrine neoplasia type 1 (MEN1) and von Hippel-Lindau disease (VHL) is of utmost importance.
- The complex nature of pNEN requires multiple medical specialities for diagnostic work-up, therapy, and follow-up; thus, the indication for surgery and the type of surgery should be discussed preoperatively in a multidisciplinary meeting.
- Some patients with pNEN might require therapy with a somatostatin analogue late after the initial surgical procedure to stabilize progression or to control hormonal excesses in metastasized disease. Because of its side effect of inducing gallstone development, cholecystectomy should be proposed to patients at the time of the initial surgery (exception: benign insulinoma).

Pre- and Perioperative Management (General Aspects)

- To avoid specific post-splenectomy infections, patients who undergo splenectomy must be vaccinated with Meningitec® and Pneumovax® at discharge or 2 weeks after the operation at the latest. If splenectomy is planned as part of the surgical procedure needed to remove pNEN, these vaccinations can be given at least 2 weeks preoperatively.
- Some studies have shown that perioperative treatment with a somatostatin analogue (e.g., 2–4 subcutaneous injections of 0.1–0.2 mg) reduces pancreatic fistula after pancreatic resection. Evidence of the effectiveness of this measure in regard to overall morbidity and mortality remains controversial; therefore, it cannot be recommended as a general rule. Its use will depend on personal preference, experience, and sometimes intraoperative conditions.

Insulin-Producing pNEN (Insulinoma)

Hallmarks

- Most insulinomas are small (<2 cm).
- Most insulinomas are benign (90 %).

---

[1] Bosman FT. WHO classification of tumors of the digestive system. Lyon: IARC Press; 2010.
[2] UICC. TNM classification of malignant tumours. 7th ed. New York: Wiley; 2011.

- Incidence: 2–4 patients/1,000,000 per year.
- 10–15 % are MEN1 associated.
- Represent approximately 25 % of pNEN.

Work-Up

Insist on:

- A properly taken family history concerning MEN1
- A proper biochemical work-up with

    - Documented neuroglycopenic symptoms during a 72-h fast test (see Chap. 8)
    - Compiled biochemical criteria obtained during the fast test: glucose ≤ 2.2 mmol/l; insulin ≥ 36 pmol/l, C-peptide ≥ 200 pmol/l, proinsulin ≥ 5 pmol/l
    - Exclusion of factitious hyperinsulinism, medication with oral sulfonylurea antidiabetics

- Preoperative localization work-up (see Chap. 9)

Pre- and Perioperative Management

- Patients with severe tendency to clinically manifest hypoglycemia should be hospitalized the day before scheduled surgery and given on a glucose infusion in order to avoid hypoglycemia during preoperative fasting.
- Preoperative information and patient consent must include all classical types of pancreatic resection (partial pancreatoduodenectomy, distal pancreatic resection, depending on preoperative localization) because the exact extent of the procedure cannot be anticipated. Even if preoperative planning suggests the possibility of a resection by "simple" enucleation, there is a possibility of intraoperative diagnosis of malignant disease or major lesion of the pancreatic duct.

Intraoperative Prerequisites

- Intraoperative ultrasound – to localize the insulinoma and ascertain its relation to the pancreatic duct and splenic vessels.
- Frozen section – to prove the resection of a neuroendocrine tumor using histopathological criteria.
- Consider using insulin monitoring (if available) and/or glucose monitoring during surgery to biochemically verify resection of the insulin-producing tumor.

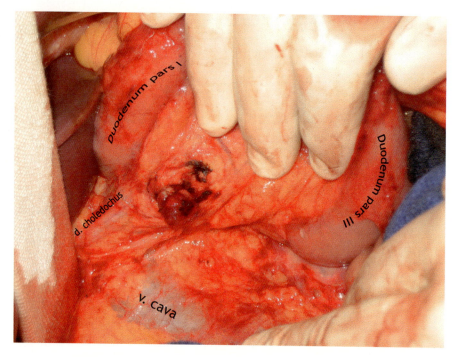

Fig. 10.1 Enucleation of a 1.5 cm insulinoma on the posterior surface of the pancreatic head in a adult

Surgical Technique

- Exposure and mobilization of head (Kocher's maneuver) and/or tail of the pancreas according to the result of the preoperative localizations studies.
- Palpation and IOUS should enable localization of the insulinoma in up to 95 % of cases.
- Enucleation

    - A simple enucleation is the procedure of choice if one can stay clear of the pancreatic duct during resection (Figs. 10.1 and 10.2).
    - Consider intraoperative secretin stimulation (2 units of secretin per kg body weight, as single intravenous bolus dose) if you are not sure whether there is a relevant lesion to the pancreatic duct or to a related contributing duct.
    - If a leak of pancreatic juice occurs on stimulation, cover the defect with a Roux-en-Y (side-to-side pancreatojejunostomy) or pursue a standard pancreatic resection (e.g., distal spleen-preserving pancreatic resection).

- If there is intraoperative suspicion of malignancy, attempt verification by frozen section and revert to an oncological resection type (right: pylorus-preserving partial pancreatoduodenectomy (PPPD), left: distal pancreatectomy).
- Never resort to "blind" resections. If you do not identify the insulinoma, close the abdomen and reevaluate diagnosis and imaging. Consider regionalization of the insulin-producing source with ASVS if not yet done.

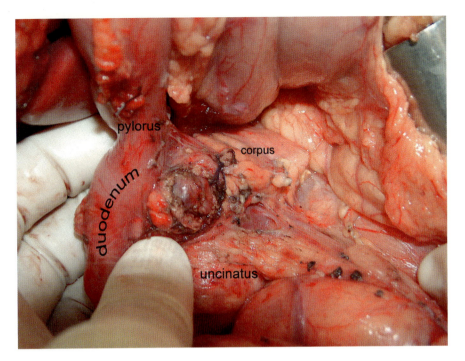

Fig. 10.2 Enucleation of a 1.5 cm insulinoma on the anterior surface of the pancreatic head in a 9-year-old child

- Laparoscopic surgery

  - Since palpation is not available, intraoperative ultrasound with a laparoscopic probe is mandatory for precise tumor localization and its topographical relation to the pancreatic duct.
  - Laparoscopic enucleation may be considered for superficially localized insulinomas that are mainly of the body and tail of the pancreas and that lack contact with major vessels or the pancreatic duct.
  - If the insulinoma lies in the tail and cannot be reasonably enucleated laparoscopically, laparoscopic distal spleen-preserving pancreatectomy may be an appropriate option.

Insulinoma (MEN1 Related)

- May be multifocal
- May be present in addition to other functioning or nonfunctioning pNEN, therefore:

  - Insist on preoperative regionalization (ASVS test, Imamura test) to ascertain the NEN responsible for hyperinsulinemia
  - In presence of multiple pNEN

- Insist on a complete biochemical work-up, including gastrin, glucagon, somatostatin, pancreatic polypeptide (PP), and chromogranin A (CrA);

include vasoactive intestinal polypeptide (VIP) only in cases with specific typical clinical symptoms.
- Plan for a resection type that meets the requirements of multiple MEN1-related NEN (usually spleen-preserving distal pancreatectomy, eventually combined with enucleation in the head).

Gastrin-Producing NEN of the Duodenum/Pancreas (Gastrinoma): Zollinger-Ellison Syndrome (ZES)

Hallmarks

- Most gastrinomas are small and located in the duodenum or pancreatic head ("gastrinoma triangle") (see Chap. 9).
- The clinical manifestations comprise recurrent (often complicated) peptic ulcer disease, chronic secretory diarrhea, and peptic esophagitis.
- All gastrinomas should be considered malignant.
- Up to 45 % of patients have lymph node involvement at diagnosis and 10 % present with liver metastasis.
- Hypergastrinemia leads to ECL-cell hyperplasia in the stomach that can cause the development of ECL-omas (type II).
- 20–30 % of gastrinomas are MEN1 associated.
- Gastrinomas represent approximately 15 % of pNEN.

Work-Up

Insist on:

- A properly taken family history concerning MEN1
- A proper clinical and biochemical work-up (see Chap. 8)

  - Evaluation for typically elevated fasting gastrin
  - Exclusion of other conditions leading to high gastrin levels:

    - Medication with proton pump inhibitors (PPIs)
    - Chronic atrophic gastritis (CAG)
    - Chronic renal insufficiency
    - *Helicobacter pylori* infection
    - Short bowel syndrome
    - Gastric outlet obstruction

  - Secretin stimulation test (see Chap. 8)
  - Biochemical screening for other potential MEN1-associated diseases

- Preoperative localization work-up (see Chap. 9)

Intraoperative Prerequisites

- Intraoperative ultrasound – to localize the gastrinoma within the pancreas
- Frozen section – to prove the resection of a neuroendocrine tumor and safe resection margins based on histopathological criteria
- Intraoperative gastroduodenoscopy – for transillumination to detect gastrinomas in the duodenal wall

Indication for Surgery

- There is general agreement that all patients with sporadic gastrinoma without evidence of hepatic metastasis and no relevant comorbidities should undergo explorative surgery with the intention to cure.

  – Arguments:

    - Up to 95 % of gastrinomas are localized intraoperatively.
    - Biochemical cure is achieved in up to 60 %.
    - Surgery prolongs disease-free survival and reduces the development of hepatic metastasis.

- Even in situations without positive localization in imaging studies, but with positive regionalization by ASVS to the duodenum/head of the pancreas, patients should be operated upon because they are very likely to have a small, resectable gastrinoma of the duodenum.

Surgical Technique

- Gastrinomas in the body or tail of the pancreas: distal pancreatectomy with splenectomy and clearance of the regional lymph nodes.
- Gastrinomas in the head of the pancreas: if locally appropriate, plan an enucleation with regional lymph node clearance and lymphadenectomy along the hepatoduodenal ligament. However, consider pylorus-preserving partial pancreatoduodenectomy (PPPPD) as an alternative.
- Proven or suspected gastrinomas of the duodenum: after complete Kocher's maneuver, localize gastrinomas by palpation and/or transillumination. Small gastrinomas can be resected in their mucosal layer after longitudinal duodenotomy in the second part of the duodenum. Larger tumors (>5 mm) should be removed with a full-thickness resection of the duodenal wall. Regional lymph node clearance and lymphadenectomy along the hepatoduodenal ligament are mandatory.

Gastrinomas (MEN1 Related)

Indication for Surgery

- This issue is and has been the topic of many discussions, with controversial attitudes on how to surgically treat MEN1 patients with ZES without evidence of a hepatic spread.
- Facts:
  - Most MEN1-associated gastrinomas are small, multiple, and located in the duodenum.
  - MEN1-associated gastrinomas tend to have a much more benign disease course than sporadic ones; this has to be carefully balanced against the morbidity of any surgical intervention.
  - After conservative surgical management (duodenotomy, local resection, and regional lymph node clearance), few patients will be biochemically cured, and a relevant part will recur since the underlying pathology in MEN1 patients is a G-cell hyperplasia in the duodenum.
  - Proponents of a Whipple procedure or PPPPD for MEN1 patients with ZES report high biochemical cure rates (>75 %).
- Attitudes in regard to indication for surgery:
  - Conservative approach: operative exploration is proposed when a localized, gastrin-producing pNEN reaches a diameter of 2 cm (higher risk of development of liver metastasis).
  - Proactive approach: operative exploration is proposed in all patients with biochemically proven ZES.

Type of Surgery

- In the absence of any randomized trials, this aspect is managed differently in different centers with great experience in endocrine surgery.
  - Conservative approach: duodenotomy, local resection of evident duodenal tumors, and regional lymph node clearance
  - Proactive approach: pylorus-preserving partial pancreatoduodenectomy (PPPPD)
- Author's comment: The final decision on extent and type of surgery will depend mainly on local skills and talent. In centers with a great experience in pancreatic surgery and low morbidity, a more radical approach may well be justified; on the other hand, in less experienced hands, a more conservative approach would be prudent.

Other Aspects

- Since hypercalcemia simulates gastrin secretion, concomitant primary hyperparathyroidism in MEN1 patients with ZES should also be addressed surgically.

Nonfunctioning pNEN

Hallmarks

- Up to 50 % of all pNEN are nonfunctioning.
- They are considered "silent" or "nonfunctioning" because they lack clinical symptoms based on a hormone excess.
- May nevertheless produce:

  - Excessive hormones that cause no overt clinical symptoms
  - Clinically relevant hormones but at levels too low to become clinically manifest

- Develop in up to 40–60 % of patients with MEN1.
- Are mostly located in pancreatic head.
- Are mostly diagnosed "incidentally" in abdominal imaging, in a work-up for unspecific abdominal discomfort, or occasionally because of obstructive symptoms (e.g., jaundice) in non-MEN1 situations.

Work-Up

- Biochemistry: CrA and pancreatic polypeptide (PP) are usually elevated.
- Fine needle aspiration (FNA) can prove the neuroendocrine character of a tumor of unknown origin.
- Biopsy can provide information concerning the differentiation and aggressiveness of the tumor (Ki67 proliferation index).
- Gastroduodenoscopy and EUS eventually combined with endoscopic FNA.

Preoperative Imaging Work-Up (See Chap. 9)

- CT/MRI for local extension and assessment of hepatic spread (usually a hypervascularized lesion) (Fig. 10.3)
- Somatostatin receptor scintigraphy (Octreoscan) (mostly positive)

Indication for Surgery

- For a non-MEN1-associated, nonfunctioning pNEN without evidence of metastasis, the treatment of choice is a standard pancreatic resection with the aim of an R0 resection. However, recent publications suggest that an observational strategy or limited resection (e.g., laparoscopic spleen-preserving distal pancreatectomy or conventional central pancreatic resection with regional lymphadenectomy)

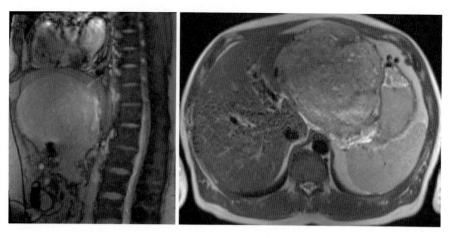

Fig. 10.3 Huge, non-functioning, well-differentiated pNEN of the pancreatic tail in a 46-year-old man with moderate, non-specific symptoms in the upper abdomen

    may be justified in patients with incidentally discovered sporadic pNEN of <2 cm in size.

- Metastatic G1 or G2 pNEN (according to the 2010 WHO classification) usually show a slow disease progression, not comparable with the course of a metastatic pancreatic adenocarcinoma. In this situation, resection of the primary tumor and surgical treatment of hepatic metastases (by resection or, e.g., radiofrequency ablation) may be justified in absence of extrahepatic disease. Such an indication should be well discussed as part of an interdisciplinary plan with oncologists and nuclear medicine specialists.

- In presence of a G3 tumor (Ki67 proliferation rate of >20 %) with a very poor prognosis, the indication for any surgical procedure should handled very restrictively.

Type of Surgery

- In non-metastatic disease, R0 resection should be attempted by classical partial pancreatoduodenectomy or distal splenopancreatectomy, depending on the localization of the tumor. Rarely, central pancreatectomy or even a total pancreatectomy might be indicated.

- In a metastatic situation with hepatic spread, the type of resection used to remove the primary tumor will also correspond to a partial pancreatoduodenectomy or distal splenopancreatectomy. Hepatic metastasis will be approached by atypical or standard types of hepatic resection or radiofrequency ablation (RFA).

- Palliative procedures could also include gastrojejunostomy to treat gastric outlet obstruction or hepatic jejunostomy to manage obstructive jaundice in cases where intraluminal stenting is impossible.

Nonfunctioning pNEN (MEN1 Related)

Hallmarks

- More than 50 % of MEN1 gene mutation carriers will develop one or more non-functioning pNEN during their lifetime.
- Nonfunctioning pNEN are a significant cause of death in MEN1 patients, accounting for approximately 15 % of the overall mortality.
- Studies have shown that surgery for nonfunctioning pNEN <2 cm in MEN1 patients is not beneficial and suggest that these patients should be followed up regularly.

Indication for Surgery

- MEN1 patients should undergo surgery in case of:
  - Nonfunctioning pNEN >2 cm
  - Nonfunctioning pNEN < 2 cm with possible radiological signs of malignancy
  - Nonfunctioning pNEN <2 cm with documented increase in diameter of >5 mm in 1 year

Types of Surgery

- Regarding the extent of resection, one should take into account that these patients may develop new pNEN during their lifetime and require further resections over time.
- For small, isolated, nonfunctioning pNEN enucleation or parenchyma, sparing distal pancreatic resection can be an option.
- For selected patients, laparoscopic spleen-preserving distal pancreatectomy can represent a valuable option.
- In case of multiple pNEN, classic distal pancreatic with or without spleen preservation represents the procedure of choice.

Very Rare Functioning pNEN (VIPoma, Glucagonoma, Somatostatinoma, PPoma)

- Are mostly malignant.
- May also secrete: serotonin, adrenocorticotropic hormone (ACTH), calcitonin, and growth hormone-releasing hormone (GHRH).

- In non-overtly metastatic disease, radical surgery (R0) should be attempted by standard oncologic pancreatic resection.
- Debulking operations to reduce the tumor load or the hormonal load should include >90 % of the tumor to be beneficial.

Complications in Pancreatic Surgery

Early Complications

- Systemic inflammatory response syndrome (SIRS)

  - Requires surveillance in an intermediate care unit or intensive care unit for 24–48 h, and eventually treatment

- Early postoperative hemorrhage

  - Intra-abdominal: generally requires operative revision
  - Intraluminal: consider endoscopic hemostasis for anastomotic bleeding (e.g., from the gastrojejunostomy)

Midterm Complications

- Delayed gastric emptying

  - Usually requires a nasogastric tube, eventually prokinetic drugs (e.g., erythromycin), and patience
  - Can be a manifestation of other intra-abdominal complications (pancreatic leak, abscess)

- Pancreatic fistula (insufficiency of a pancreatojejunostomy or of the pancreatic stump closure in distal pancreatectomy)

  - Monitor quality and quantity of the fluids drained every day.
  - Regularly measure amylase and bilirubin in the fluids.
  - In manifest fistula:

    - Keep drainages in place.
    - Fasting, somatostatin analogue, and parenteral nutrition.
    - Interventional percutaneous drainage of insufficiently drained intra-abdominal fluid collections.
    - Very rarely, total pancreatectomy might be needed in cases of progressive multiorgan failure.

- Secondary intra-abdominal hemorrhage from pseudoaneurysms of major visceral vessels (mostly from the stump of the gastroduodenal artery or the hepatic arteries)

  - Usually a consequence of pancreatic fistula
  - Has a high mortality
  - Be alarmed by a "sentinel bleed" in the drain fluid and investigate immediately with contrast-enhanced CT
  - Preferably consider early interventional coiling or stenting
  - If not possible, operative revision

- Bile leakage from bilioenteric anastomosis

  - If early postoperative (<48 h), consider operative revision.
  - If later in the postoperative course:

    - Keep drains in place.
    - Evaluate temporary percutaneous transhepatic drainage/stenting.

Pearls and Pitfalls
Pearls

- pNENs are a fascinating tumor group; every single tumor has a unique clinical presentation and requires an individualized work-up and a "custom-tailored" therapeutic approach
- An incomplete preoperative biochemical work-up lacking specific preoperative marker levels may compromise the postoperative oncologic follow-up

Pitfalls

- No medical discipline can treat pNEN single-handedly! pNEN treatment requires multidisciplinary team work at its best! Diagnostic work-up, therapy, and follow-up involve endocrinologists, surgeons, radiologists, nuclear medicine specialists, histopathologists, and oncologists; therefore, the indication for surgery and the type of procedure should be discussed preoperatively as part of a coherent treatment plan by an interdisciplinary board
- An inappropriate work-up concerning MEN1 can be a missed chance to recognize other MEN1-related diseases in a patient and a whole kindred

Further Reading

Akerstrom G, Falconi M, Kianmanesh R, Ruszniewski P, Plockinger U. ENETS Consensus Guidelines for the Standards of Care in Neuroendocrine Tumors: pre- and perioperative therapy in patients with neuroendocrine tumors. Neuroendocrinology. 2009;90(2):203–8.

Delle FG, Kwekkeboom DJ, Van CE, Rindi G, Kos-Kudla B, Knigge U, et al. ENETS consensus guidelines for the management of patients with gastroduodenal neoplasms. Neuroendocrinology. 2012;95(2):74–87.

Falconi M, Bartsch DK, Eriksson B, Kloppel G, Lopes JM, O'Connor JM, et al. ENETS consensus guidelines for the management of patients with digestive neuroendocrine neoplasms of the digestive system: well-differentiated pancreatic non-functioning tumors. Neuroendocrinology. 2012;95(2):120–34.

Jensen RT, Cadiot G, Brandi ML, de Herder WW, Kaltsas G, Komminoth P, et al. ENETS Consensus Guidelines for the management of patients with digestive neuroendocrine neoplasms: functional pancreatic endocrine tumor syndromes. Neuroendocrinology. 2012;95(2):98–119.

Oberg K, Eriksson B. Endocrine tumours of the pancreas. Best Pract Res Clin Gastroenterol. 2005;19(5):753–81.

Ramage JK, Ahmed A, Ardill J, Bax N, Breen DJ, Caplin ME, et al. Guidelines for the management of gastroenteropancreatic neuroendocrine (including carcinoid) tumours (NETs). Gut. 2012;61(1):6–32.

Chapter 11
Gastrointestinal Neuroendocrine Tumor (NET) Surgery

Per Hellman and Peter Stålberg

Gastrointestinal Neuroendocrine Tumors (NETs)

Definition

- GI NETs arise from stomach, duodenum, small intestine, appendix, large bowel, and appendix.
- GI NETs arise from differentiated endocrine cells in the mucosa.
- Formerly divided into foregut (stomach, duodenum, pancreas), midgut (small intestine, appendix, and cecum), and hindgut carcinoids (large bowel except cecum and rectum).
- The biological properties vary according to organ of origin.
- The latest WHO definition of NET does not consider the organ of origin instead a common definition is used that is based on factors such as Ki67 index or mitotic index and size.

Well-differentiated neuroendocrine tumor: size <2 cm and a Ki67 index <3 %
Moderately differentiated neuroendocrine tumor: size >2 cm and a Ki67 index >3 %
Poorly differentiated neuroendocrine cancer (NEC): Ki67 index >20 %

P. Hellman, MD, PhD (✉) • P. Stålberg, MD, PhD
Department of Surgical Sciences,
Uppsala University, Uppsala
SE-751 85, Sweden
e-mail: per.hellman@surgsci.uu.se

J.C. Watkinson, D.M. Scott-Coombes (eds.), *Tips and Tricks in Endocrine Surgery*,
DOI 10.1007/978-1-4471-2146-6_11, © Springer-Verlag London 2014

Epidemiology

- Overall annual incidence 2.5–5 per 100,000 people per year but much higher prevalence of ≈ 35 per 100,000.
- Most common are small intestinal NET (best known as midgut carcinoids).

Gastric NETs

Definition

- Arising from the enterochromaffin (EC) cells in the gastric mucosa
- Type I – polyps, in atrophic gastritis, high gastric pH, and high gastrin levels
- Type II – polyps/small tumours, secondary to small (<1 cm) gastrinoma, low gastric pH, and high gastrin (Zollinger-Ellison)
- Type III – Tumors (>1–2 cm), low gastrin, and larger tumors

Presentation

- Usually found at gastroscopy for vague symptoms.
- Duodenal, ectopic, HP negative, or multiple ulcers are suspicious for gastrinoma.
- Bleeding and discomfort for type III. Sometimes (rare) histamine release, giving atypical carcinoid syndrome with pulmonary obstruction.

Investigations

- Endoscopy with measurements of pH in gastric juice and multiple biopsies
- Endoscopic ultrasound for assessment of invasive depth
- CT, somatostatin receptor scintigraphy, or ^{68}Ga-DOTATOC PET for evaluation of metastases (usually type III, rarely type II) (see Chap. 9)

Medical Management

- Type I – vitamin B12.
- Type II – proton pump inhibitor.
- Somatostatin analogue may in rare cases be used in type I or II.

Indications for Surgery

Absolute Indications

- Visualized type II gastric NET (gastrinoma)
- Type III gastric NET
- Type I >1 cm

Relative Indications

- Type I <1 cm or multiple small (polypectomy or rarely Billroth II gastric resection)

Tips for Surgery

- Local excision of polyps may be performed by several different methods (simple classical polypectomy, suction technique, etc.).

Complications and Outcomes

A summary of complications is given in Table 11.1.

Table 11.1 Gastric NETs: summary of complications

Early complications	Intermediate complications	Late complications
Bleeding, perforation	Leakage, abscesses	Recurrence

Pearls and Pitfalls
Pearls

- Important to check gastrin pre- and postoperatively
- Type II may be part of MEN1

Pitfalls

- Localize gastrinoma before surgery. Use PET, SRS, etc.
- If Ki67 >20 %, classified as NEC – should not be operated initially

Duodenal NETs

Definition

- Majority in first or second part of duodenum. Rare (1–3 % of all GI NETs).
- Usually small (<2 cm) and submucosal.
- Rarely carcinoid syndrome.
- Functional (gastrin- or somatostatin) or nonfunctional.
- Gastrinoma may be part of MEN1.

Presentation

- Gastrinoma – signs for type II gastric NETs or as part of MEN1
- Somatostatinoma associated with NF1 (neurofibromatosis type 1) and gall stones
  Periampullary localization

Investigations

- Gastrin, chromogranin A (high in gastrinoma, normal in others)
- Endoscopy (ulcer, location) with measurements of pH in gastric juice
- CT, MRT, SRS, etc., low sensitivity unless tumors >5–7 mm
- Endoscopic ultrasound to investigate location, involvement of pancreatic head, lymph nodes, depth of invasion

Medical Management

- Proton pump inhibitor for gastrinoma

Indications for Surgery

Absolute Indications

- If gastrinoma is found – treat before lymph node metastases occur.

Relative Indications

- Also in presence of metastases, surgery may be palliative.

Table 11.2 Duodenal NETs: summary of complications

Early complications	Intermediate complications	Late complications
Bleeding, perforation	Leakage, abscesses	Recurrence

Tips for Surgery

Operative:

- Polypectomy, transduodenal excision, duodenal resection, or pancreaticoduodenectomy may be used.

Complications and Outcomes

A summary of complications is given in Table 11.2.

Pearls and Pitfalls
Pearls

- Duodenal gastrinoma has a good prognosis and may be left unresected and treated with PPI if not localized

Pitfalls

- Check for inherited disease! MEN1, NF1

Small Intestinal NETs

Definition

- Arising from the enterochromaffin (EC) cells in the small intestinal submucosa.
- Peak age of diagnosis is 60–70 years of age.
- Submucosal and often antimesenteric. Small (0.5–2 cm).

Presentation

- 30–40 % present at emergency surgery for bowel obstruction.
- 20 % present after work-up for unknown liver metastases.
- May be found incidentally during surgery for something else.

Fig. 11.1 Typical CT scan demonstrating fibrosis around mesenteric lymph node metastasis in small intestinal NET

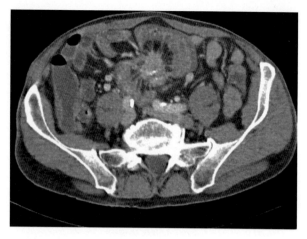

- Typical symptoms are flushing, diarrhea, and food intolerance.
- 30 % have multiple primary tumors.
- Commonly associated with marked fibrosis around mesenteric nodal metastases and cause shortening of mesentery and kinking of small bowel.

Investigations

- 5-HIAA (hydroxyindoleacetic acid) in 24-h urine is diagnostic.
- CgA is often raised but less specific (also high in renal failure, treatment with PPI).
- Typical CT scan with pathognomonic pattern in intestinal mesentery, often combined with liver metastases (Fig. 11.1).

Medical Management

- Check for concomitant carcinoid heart disease (tricuspid valve insufficiency, right-sided heart failure).
- Somatostatin analogues, initially 100–200 µg Sandostatin® three times daily, followed by monthly intramuscular injection of long-acting version.
- Supplementation with pancreatic enzymes may be needed when somatostatin analogues are given.
- Selected cases may use interferon-alpha (IntronA®) three times per week.
- For diarrhea – loperamide or other similar agents may be useful.
- Radiation therapy by ^{177}Lu-labeled octreotide may be given usually maximum four times to spare renal function in cases with liver and skeletal metastases.

Indications for Surgery

Absolute Indications

- Obstruction, also in cases with subacute obstruction.
- To remove primary tumor.
- To remove mesenteric lymph node metastases (sometimes resect and leave the upper portion if major vessels are involved).
- Liver metastases – if maximum around 5, also if bilateral, resection may be performed.
- Surgery – performed as liver embolization, with particles or radiation, if multiple bilateral liver metastases.
- Radiofrequency or microwave ablation of liver metastases is an alternative for smaller number and/or growing metastases even in the presence of many metastases.

Relative Indications

- Long-standing abdominal pain without obvious obstruction. To rule out incipient intestinal ischemia.

Tips for Surgery

Preoperative:
- Check for carcinoid heart disease with echocardiogram.
- Temporarily omit interferon alpha – it may cause leucopenia masking postoperative complications.
- Malnourished patients should be given preoperative nutritional therapy.

Operative:
- All patients should have preoperative protection with Sandostatin (e.g., 500 µg in 500 ml NaCl, infusion rate 50–100 ml/h).
- Resection of primary tumor is often easy, while mesenteric metastases may be stuck to the retroperitoneum or extending upwards beneath duodenum and pancreas and encompassing the mesenteric vessels.
- Resection of the mesenteric metastasis may be performed – better to leave intestinal length rather than perform dangerous surgery possibly leading to short bowel.
- Lift the whole intestinal mesentery by dissecting from behind to the level of horizontal duodenum.

Table 11.3 Small intestinal NETs: summary of complications

Early complications	Intermediate complications	Late complications
Bleeding	Anastomosis leakage	Obstruction

- Liver metastases may be atypically locally resected with minimal margin as long as the tumor capsule is intact – or treated preoperatively with RFA.
- Intraoperative ultrasound often reveals multiple metastases, more than anticipated from preoperative work-up.

  Postoperative:

- Continue Sandostatin infusion until the 500 μg is finished (10 h at 50 ml/h).
- Reinsert interferon alpha 2–3 weeks postoperatively (if the patient takes the drug).

Complications and Outcomes

A summary of complications is given in Table 11.3.

Pearls and Pitfalls

Pearls

- Preoperative Sandostatin infusion!
- Thorough examination of CT scans to accurately plan the mesenteric approach

Pitfalls

- Check for carcinoid heart disease
- Devascularization of mesenteric vessels
- Malnourished patient

Appendiceal NETs

Definition

- 15–20 % of all GI NETs.
- 50–75 % of all appendiceal tumors are NET.
- Usually in the tip.
- Mean age 36 years.
- May be divided into pure NET, tubular, or adenocarcinoid (mixed adenocarcinoma and endocrine).

Presentation

- Usually as appendicitis and after appendicectomy
- No carcinoid syndrome

Investigations

- Pathology: Size, invasion into mesoappendix, angioinvasion, perineural growth, lymph node involvement, goblet cells – all should be carefully examined for.

Medical Management

- None, except for adenocarcinoids – should be treated as adenocarcinoma in colon.

Indications for Surgery

- Reoperation with right hemicolectomy and lymph node clearance if size >2 cm, non-radical excision especially at the appendiceal base, signs of angio- or perineural invasion.
- Peritonectomy and intraoperative treatment with warm chemotherapy may be needed in goblet cell appendiceal NETs or adenocarcinoids.

Tips for Surgery

Preoperative:

- Rarely express somatostatin receptors, but if so future treatment may be easier – therefore check with somatostatin receptor scintigraphy (SRS) or ^{68}Ga-DOTATOC PET for expression.
- Rarely secrete CgA but should be checked preoperatively to be used as biomarker.

Operative:

- If signs of goblet cells or peritoneal carcinomatosis – extended surgery with peritonectomy or intraoperative chemotherapy may be performed.

Postoperative:

- Follow-up difficult due to few biomarkers (e.g., SRS or CgA, see above).

Table 11.4 Appendiceal NETs: summary of complications

Early complications	Intermediate complications	Late complications
Bleeding	Leakage	Recurrence, liver metastases

Complications and Outcomes

A summary of complications is given in Table 11.4.

Pearls and Pitfalls
Pearls

- Most often cured by appendicectomy alone

Pitfalls

- Signs of goblet cells, adenocarcinoid should be aggressively treated

Large Bowel NETs

Definition

- From ascending to sigmoid colon
- Same cell type as in small intestine
- More aggressive than small intestinal NETs (Fig. 11.2)

Presentation

- Usually as adenocarcinoma from colon
- Rarely carcinoid syndrome

Investigations

- CT, barium enema, colonoscopy, or colon CT are useful.
- SRS – since they may express somatostatin receptors (important in follow-up/ treatment option).

Medical Management

- Cases with Ki67 >20 % (NEC – not rare) are treated with chemotherapy.

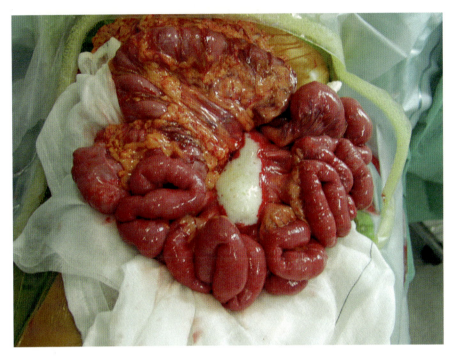

Fig. 11.2 Large inoperable mesenteric mass of fibrosis and tumor in small intestinal NET

Indications for Surgery

Absolute Indications

- Obstruction, bleeding – also if metastases

Relative Indications

- If initial massive liver metastases, ^{177}Lu therapy may downstage and lead to operable disease if SRS is positive.

Tips for Surgery

Experienced colorectal surgeon.

Complications and Outcomes

A summary of complications is given in Table 11.5.

Table 11.5 Large bowel NETs: summary of complications

Early complications	Intermediate complications	Late complications
Bleeding	Leakage, abscesses	Recurrence

Pearls and Pitfalls
Pearls

- Presentation as colonic adenocarcinoma

Pitfalls

- In case of metastases downstaging may be possible

Rectal NETs

Definition

- 15–20 % of all GI NETs.
- Immunostaining for GLP (glucagon-like peptide) or PSA. Certain L cells may be present.

Presentation

- >50 % have no symptoms, often incidental finding – remainder bleeding, pain, and discomfort
- No carcinoid syndrome
- Generally low Ki67 (<1 %)

Investigations

- Chromogranin A is often normal (but may be high and should be checked).
- CEA and PSA are potential biomarkers.
- Rectal ultrasound and MRT to check for pathological lymph nodes and invasion in rectal wall.
- Somatostatin receptor scintigraphy in case of metastases is useful.

Medical Management

- None, unless there are metastases. If so – ^{177}Lu therapy may be effective if positive SRS.

Table 11.6 Rectal NETs: summary of complications

Early complications	Intermediate complications	Late complications
Bleeding	Abscesses	Recurrence, pain

Indications for Surgery

- <1 cm – local excision (polypectomy); 1–2 cm TEM (transanal mucosal excision); >2 cm TME (total mesorectal excision) and anterior resection.
- In case of metastases, ^{68}Lu therapy may induce tumor reduction allowing surgery.

Tips for Surgery

- Work-up is essential to find signs of rectal wall invasion or pelvic lymph nodes, which governs type of surgery.

Complications and Outcomes

A summary of complications is given in Table 11.6.

Pearls and Pitfalls
Pearls

- Majority (>90 %) cured after simple polypectomy

Pitfalls

- If not properly worked up preoperatively and signs of invasion or local spread neglected, high risk for distant metastases later in the course

Further Reading

Åkerström G, Hellman P. Carcinoid neoplasms. In: Bland KI, Büchler MW, Csendes A, Garden OJ, Sarr MG, Wong J, editors. General surgery. Berlin: Springer; 2009. p. 1709–18.

Cashin P, Nygren P, Hellman P, Granberg D, Mahteme H. A survey of appendiceal adenocarcinoids with peritoneal carcinomatosis: Overall survival, pharmacological drug resistance and their histopathology. Clin Colorectal Cancer. 2011;20:108–12.

Delle Fave G, Capurso G, Milione M, Panzuto F. Endocrine tumours of the stomach. Best Pract Res Clin Gastroenterol. 2005;19:659–73.

Norlén O, Stålberg P, Eriksson J, Hedberg J, Hessman O, Tienssu-Janson E, Hellman P, Åkerström G. Long-term results of surgery for small intestinal neuroendocrine tumors at a tertiary referral center. World J Surg. 2012;36(6):1414–31.

Stinner B, Rothmund M. Neuroendocrine tumours (carcinoids) of the appendix. Best Pract Res Clin Gastroenterol. 2005;19:729–38.

Vogelsang H, Siewert JR. Endocrine tumours of the hindgut. Best Pract Res Clin Gastroenterol. 2005;19:739–52.

Part III
Thyroid

Chapter 12
Assessment of Goiter

Helen Cocks and Kristien Boelaert

Definition

- Goiter is a nonspecific term for enlargement of the thyroid gland.
- Goiters are characterized by excessive growth and structural and/or functional transformation of one or several areas within the normal thyroid tissue.
- Goiters can be diffused or nodular (containing a single or multiple nodules).
- Goiters may occur sporadically and are endemic in areas of iodine deficiency.
- Most goiters can be treated conservatively after thyroid dysfunction and malignancy have been ruled out.

WHO Definition

A thyroid whose lateral lobes have a volume greater than the terminal phalanges of the thumb of the person being examined.

H. Cocks, MD, MBChB, FRCS (✉)
Department of Otolaryngology, City Hospitals Sunderland NHS Trust,
Kayll Road, Sunderland SR4 7TP, UK
e-mail: helen.cocks@chsft.nhs.uk

K. Boelaert, MD, PhD, MRCP
Department of Endocrinology,
University Hospital Birmingham, Birmingham, UK

Centre for Endocrinology, Diabetes and Metabolism,
Institute of Biomedical Research,
School of Clinical and Experimental Medicine,
University of Birmingham,
Birmingham B15 2TH, UK

J.C. Watkinson, D.M. Scott-Coombes (eds.), *Tips and Tricks in Endocrine Surgery*,
DOI 10.1007/978-1-4471-2146-6_12, © Springer-Verlag London 2014

Prevalence

- Goiters are common; the Whickham Survey of a representative sample of the adult population in the UK reported a prevalence of palpable goiter of 15.5 % (Tunbridge et al. 1977). A follow-up study 20 years later found the incidence of goiter in the surviving females had fallen from 26 to 10 %, confirming the observation that goiters may regress as people get older.
- When ultrasonographic determination of thyroid volume is undertaken, the frequency of goiter is up to 25 %.
- The Framingham study in the USA estimated solitary nodules to be present in 4.6 %, and the lifetime risk of developing a nodule was estimated at between 5 and 10 % (Vander et al. 1968). Fifty percent of subjects have thyroid nodules at autopsy, a finding confirmed by ultrasound studies.
- Up to 50 % of subjects with a solitary palpable nodule or a diffusely enlarged thyroid gland actually have multiple nodules when investigated by ultrasound.
- Goiters are 4–10 times more common in females than in males.
- Thyroid cancer usually presents with thyroid enlargement. Thyroid cancer is rare accounting for approximately 1 % of all new malignancies and 0.5 % of all cancer deaths.
- The incidence of thyroid cancer in euthyroid patients presenting with goiter to a tertiary referral center is estimated between 5 and 10 %. Solitary nodules are usually dominant nodules in a multinodular goiter but if truly solitary carry a 20 % risk of malignancy.

Presentation

- Patients with thyroid enlargement present both to the endocrinologist and to the surgeon. Patients referred to the surgeon are usually euthyroid having presented with a neck lump. Many are sent on the 2-week referral pathway although they have no worrying features.
- Some patients are referred with overt symptoms and signs of thyroid dysfunction, and it is important to recognize these. Patients with thyroid dysfunction should primarily be managed by endocrinologists.
- Patients with thyrotoxicosis, due to toxic nodular or Graves' disease may be referred for consideration of total thyroidectomy if hyperthyroidism is poorly controlled medically, if they have developed significant adverse effects to antithyroid drugs, or if they have significant thyroid eye disease preventing the administration of radioiodine.

The majority of thyroid disease is benign. The challenge of the clinician is to identify those patients who have malignant disease so that they may receive timely, effective treatment.

Table 12.1 World Health
Organization classification
of goiter by examination

Classification	Finding
0	No goiter palpable or visible
1a	Goiter detected by palpation only
1b	Goiter palpable and visible with neck extended
2	Goiter visible with neck in normal position
3	Large goiter visible from a distance

Clinical Evaluation

In most cases thyroid glands harboring malignancy are clinically indistinguishable from those that do not, and there is substantial variation among clinicians in evaluating nodules.

Symptoms and signs are rarely diagnostic of thyroid malignancy.

History

- *Time course*: It is important to determine the rate of growth. A rapidly growing goiter may indicate malignancy. A sudden appearance of a nodule can be seen following the rupture of follicles and hemorrhage into a nodule.
- *Pain*: Discomfort is uncommon but can be a feature of benign inflammatory disease or hemorrhage into a cyst. In malignant disease, there may be referred pain to the ear.
- *Pressure*: The patient may complain of pressure symptoms in the neck. It is important to determine whether there is any dysphagia or dyspnea which may indicate esophageal or tracheal compression. This may occur with large (retrosternal) goiter or with thyroid cancer.
- *Stridor*: This can result either from extreme tracheal compression due to a large multinodular goiter or from recurrent laryngeal nerve palsy; the latter is usually associated with malignancy but is not diagnostic of it.
- *Change in voice*: May result from recurrent laryngeal nerve palsy.
- *Ionizing radiation exposure*: Particularly to the head and neck as a child increases the risk of thyroid cancer. Epidemiological studies have observed increased rates of childhood papillary thyroid cancer in Belarus and Ukraine following the Chernobyl nuclear reactor accident in 1986 (Hegedus et al. 2003; Hegedus 2004; Pacini et al. 1997).
- *Place of emigration*: (if relevant) Iodine deficiency confers a higher risk of goiter and is associated with follicular thyroid cancer.
- *Family history*: A family history of thyroid disease is common. A family history of malignancy conveys an increased risk.
- *Gender*: Men presenting with thyroid enlargement have significantly higher rates of malignancy compared with women.
- *Drug history*: The intake of antithyroid drugs (carbimazole, propylthiouracil), thyroxine, lithium, and also iodine-containing drugs or foods should be recorded (see Table 12.1.).

Examination

There is considerable inter- and intra-observer variation regarding size and morphology of the thyroid gland.

- The physical examination should focus on inspection of the neck and upper thorax and palpation of the goiter to determine its size and nodularity. The examination should ideally be done with the patient swallowing gulps of water and the head tilted slightly backwards.
- Determine character of the thyroid gland: smooth or nodular surface, single or multiple nodules, and soft or hard. Determine if the lower limit of the thyroid gland can be palpated. Get the patient to extend their neck to see if you can get to the lower limit.
- Determine indicators of compression (stridor, Pemberton's sign, thyroid cork and Berry's sign – see Chap. 20: Surgery for Retrosternal Goiter). Assess the neck and supraclavicular area for enlarged lymph nodes.
- Assess if the thyroid gland is fixed or mobile. Mobility on swallowing may be lost in Riedel's thyroiditis (chronic form of thyroiditis associated with extensive fibrosis) or in anaplastic carcinoma.
- Assess vocal cord mobility.

Laboratory Investigations

- *Serum thyrotropin (TSH) concentration*. This should be measured in all patients with thyroid enlargement (British Thyroid Association (BTA) and American Thyroid Association (ATA) guidelines) (British Thyroid Association and Royal College of Physicians 2007; Cooper et al. 2009).
- If *TSH* is low, then serum *free triiodothyronine (fT3)* and *free thyroxine (fT4) concentrations* are required to exclude overt hyperthyroidism (raised serum fT4 and fT3 concentrations) or T3 toxicosis (raised serum fT3 concentration alone).
- If *TSH* is raised, then overt hypothyroidism must be excluded (low serum fT4 concentration).
- Thyroid dysfunction is rarely associated with malignant disease.
- *Thyroid autoantibodies*. Microsomal, thyroid peroxidase, or TSH receptor antibodies are found in about 10 % of the general population and may coexist with goiter. Levels are elevated in the majority of patients with autoimmune thyroiditis and Graves' disease. Their presence can alter the interpretation of FNAC and therefore are of importance to the cytopathologist.
- *Calcitonin*. Routine use is not recommended, but it should be performed if medullary thyroid cancer is suspected.
- *Thyroglobulin*. There is no role for the routine measurement of serum thyroglobulin in the initial evaluation of thyroid nodules; however, it is used as a

tumor marker following total thyroidectomy and radioiodine ablation for differentiated thyroid cancer.

Flow-Volume Loop Studies

- These provide a sensitive and specific measure of upper airway obstruction and thus provide functional information superior to that obtained from routine chest and neck radiography.

Diagnostic Imaging

Ultrasonography (*USS*) is the most widely used imaging technique in the evaluation of goiters.

- USS is highly sensitive and can detect non-palpable nodules. There is a risk of identifying clinically insignificant nodules resulting in unnecessary investigations and associated anxiety for the patient (Hegedus et al. 2003; Hegedus 2001).
- USS can estimate the size of nodules and the goiter volume which may be useful in monitoring and assessment of response to treatment.
- Some USS characteristics are associated with an increased cancer risk and can be useful when used in conjunction with other investigations. For example, in complex cysts, the appearance of the cyst wall can be described, and solid areas can be targeted for aspiration. Microcalcifications can be seen on USS with coarse calcification usually reflecting colloid nodules and finer calcifications seen in papillary thyroid cancers.
- USS is effective at identifying suspicious nodes in 20–30 % of patients with papillary thyroid cancer. It is recommended that a fine needle aspiration of ultrasonographically suspicious lesions is performed.

Scintigraphy

- This is a historic investigation for the evaluation of goiters and nodules. It is helpful in assessment of the function of nodules. It has been largely superseded by ultrasonography and fine needle aspiration cytology.
- Hot (functional) nodules can be distinguished from cold (nonfunctional) nodules (Hegedus et al. 2003; British Thyroid Association and Royal College of Physicians 2007).
- The risk of malignancy in cold nodules is reported as high as 8–25 %.

Table 12.2 Ultrasound characteristics raising suspicion for malignancy

USS characteristics suspicious for malignancy
Hypoechogenicity
Solid nodules
Microcalcifications
Irregular margins
Increased intranodular flow (Doppler)
Increased ratio of anterior/posterior dimensions in transverse and longitudinal views (More tall than wide)
Evidence of invasion
Evidence of regional lymphadenopathy

CT and MRI

- CT and MRI are not used routinely but may have a role in the assessment of retrosternal goiter and in malignancy where there is extensive nodal involvement or local invasion or when hemoptysis reported.
- When malignancy is suspected or confirmed, CT should be without the use of iodinated contrast medium since this can block iodine uptake by the gland for some time and prevent the use of radioactive iodine as an adjuvant in the treatment of differentiated thyroid cancer.

FDG-PET

- May be used in the follow-up of patients with proven differentiated thyroid cancer. It currently has no place in the routine evaluation of patients with goiter.

Fine Needle Aspiration Cytology (FNAC)

- This remains the gold standard first-line investigation of any thyroid nodule (BTA and ATA guidelines) (British Thyroid Association and Royal College of Physicians 2007; Cooper et al. 2009). Solitary nodules and dominant (largest) nodules in multinodular goiter are targeted. Nodules over 10 mm in diameter and those with any suspicious features should also be targeted (Cooper et al. 2009).
- It has low complication rates, is inexpensive, and easy to learn.
- Has been shown to reduce the number of patients requiring surgery by 35–75 % and to improve the yield of malignancy at thyroidectomy threefold (Castro and Gharib 2005).
- Has been evaluated in several studies with sensitivities between 65 and 98 % and specificity between 72 and 100 % (Sherman 2003; Gharib and Goellner 1993).
- The use of USS increases sensitivity and specificity compared with palpation-guided FNAC by reducing the number of non-diagnostic aspirates (Hegedus

Table 12.3 Thyroid FNA diagnostic categories and action as per BTA guidelines

BTA diagnostic category	Description	Action
THY 1	Non-diagnostic	Repeat FNAC – USS guided preferable
		Close observation
		Consider surgery if solid nodule, if worrying USS signs or recurrent cyst
THY 2	Non-neoplastic	Repeat aspirate after 3–6 months
THY 3	Follicular lesion	Indicates follicular lesion (*see* Chap. 3 *for*
	Other worrying lesions that do not fit Thy2 or 4	*more details on the indeterminate thyroid lesion*)
THY4	Suspicious for malignancy	Surgery usually indicated for suspected cancer
	DTC, MTC, anaplastic, lymphoma	Further investigations maybe required
THY 5	Diagnostic for malignancy	Surgery for DTC, MTC
	DTC, MTC, anaplastic, lymphoma	Radiotherapy ± chemotherapy for anaplastic cancers and lymphoma

DTC differentiated thyroid cancer, *MTC* medullary thyroid cancer

et al. 2003; Hegedus 2004). Ultrasound findings can be used in conjunction with FNAC results, thereby improving diagnostic accuracy (see Table 12.2).

- The clinical usefulness of FNAC depends on the sampling of adequate material, and approximately 15 % of all specimens remain non-diagnostic. This is mainly due to inadequate sampling that can be improved with repeat biopsy (Castro and Gharib 2005).
- Cysts should be completely aspirated and any residual mass re-aspirated immediately. If aspiration results in no residual mass, then one can be less concerned (British Thyroid Association and Royal College of Physicians 2007).
- Cytological results from FNAC should be reported according to the current BTA and ATA guidance as shown in Table 12.3. This also displays the action that should be taken following each cytological diagnosis.
- All cases in which there is a definite or suspected diagnosis of neoplasia or those where there are discrepancies between clinical, radiological, and cytological findings should be discussed at the thyroid multidisciplinary team meeting (British Thyroid Association and Royal College of Physicians 2007).

References

British Thyroid Association and Royal College of Physicians. Guidelines for the management of thyroid cancer. 2007. www.british-thyroid-association.org.
Castro MR, Gharib H. Continuing controversies in the management of thyroid nodules. Ann Intern Med. 2005;142:926–31.

Cooper DS, Doherty GM, Haugen BR, et al. Revised American Thyroid Association Management Guidelines for patients with Thyroid nodules and differentiated thyroid cancer. Thyroid. 2009; 19(11):1167–214.

Gharib H, Goellner JR. Fine-needle aspiration biopsy of the thyroid: an appraisal. Ann Intern Med. 1993;118:282–9.

Hegedus L. Thyroid ultrasound. Endocrinol Metab Clin North Am. 2001;30:339–60.

Hegedus L. Clinical practice. The thyroid nodule. N Engl J Med. 2004;351:1764–71.

Hegedus L, Bonnema SJ, Bennedbaek FN. Management of simple nodular goiter: current status and future perspectives. Endocr Rev. 2003;24:102–32.

Pacini F, Vorontsova T, Demidchik E, et al. Post Chernobyl thyroid carcinoma in Belarus children and adolescents:comparison with naturally occurring thyroid carcinoma in Italy and France. J Endocrinol Metab. 1997;82(11):3563–9.

Sherman SI. Thyroid carcinoma. Lancet. 2003;361:501–11.

Tunbridge WM, Evered DC, Hall R, et al. The spectrum of thyroid disease in a community: the Whickham survey. Clin Endocrinol. 1977;7:481–93.

Vander JB, Gaston EA, Dawber TR. The significance of nontoxic thyroid nodules. Final report of a 15-year study of the incidence of thyroid malignancy. Ann Intern Med. 1968;69:537–40.

Chapter 13
Surgery for Benign Thyroid Disease

Sharan Jayaram, Kristien Boelaert, and Ian D. Hay

Introduction

- Enlargement of the thyroid gland (goiter) is the most common endocrine disorder worldwide; the vast majority are benign.
- There are well-defined clinical guidelines for surgical management of thyroid malignancies (Cooper et al. 2009; British Thyroid Association and Royal College of Physicians 2007) but no universally accepted surgical protocol exists for benign thyroid disease.

Classification of Benign Thyroid Pathology

- Goiters can be classified based on the presence (toxic goiters) or absence (nontoxic goiters) of thyroid hyperfunction, as well as the presence of one (solitary) or multiple (multinodular) nodules.

S. Jayaram
Department of Otolaryngology, Head and Neck Surgery,
University Hospital Birmingham,
Birmingham, UK

K. Boelaert, MD, PhD, MRCP (✉)
Department of Endocrinology, University Hospital Birmingham,
Birmingham, UK

Centre for Endocrinology, Diabetes and Metabolism, Institute of Biomedical Research,
School of Clinical and Experimental Medicine, University of Birmingham,
Birmingham B15 2TH, UK
e-mail: k.boelaert@bham.ac.uk

I.D. Hay
Division of Endocrinology, Diabetes, Metabolism, and Nutrition, Mayo Clinic,
Rochester, MN, USA

J.C. Watkinson, D.M. Scott-Coombes (eds.), *Tips and Tricks in Endocrine Surgery*,
DOI 10.1007/978-1-4471-2146-6_13, © Springer-Verlag London 2014

Table 13.1 Classification of benign thyroid pathology

Simple(nontoxic) goiter	Multinodular
	Solitary thyroid nodule
	Follicular adenoma
	Thyroid cyst
Toxic goiter	Diffuse (Graves' disease)
	Toxic multinodular (Plummer's disease)
	Solitary toxic adenoma
Inflammatory goiter	Acute suppurative thyroiditis
	Subacute (painless) lymphocytic, including postpartum thyroiditis
	Subacute (painful) granulomatous or De Quervain's thyroiditis
	Chronic lymphocytic or Hashimoto's autoimmune thyroiditis
	Invasive fibrous (Riedel's) thyroiditis
Developmental conditions	Thyroglossal duct cyst
	Ectopic thyroid (lingual)
Rare causes of goiter	Amyloid goiter
	Dyshormonogenetic goiter
	Drug induced (lithium, amiodarone)

- Multinodular goiter (MNG) is the most common benign pathology affecting the thyroid gland (Table 13.1).

Simple (Nontoxic) Goiter

- *Multinodular goiter* may affect up to 500–600 million people worldwide (Matovinevic 1983).

  - May be sporadic, endemic (in areas of iodine-deficiency), or, rarely, familial.
  - Majority of patients are euthyroid and asymptomatic; a slow, gradual (10–20 % per year) increase in volume is usual.

- *Follicular adenoma* is a benign, encapsulated, noninvasive follicular cell neoplasm that may display only very subtle histopathologic differences from adjacent thyroid parenchyma.

  - Pathological variants include Hürthle cell adenoma, hyalinizing trabecular adenoma, and atypical follicular adenoma.
  - Since follicular adenomas cannot be differentiated from carcinomas using fine needle aspiration biopsy (FNAB), the term "follicular neoplasm" is used, and surgical excision is required to establish a definite diagnosis.

- *Thyroid cysts* can be easily identified using thyroid ultrasonography.

  - They may be caused by a variety of etiologies (infectious, inflammatory, degenerative, neoplastic), although cystic degeneration within a multinodular goiter is the most common cause.

Toxic Goiter

- *Graves' disease* is a common autoimmune disorder characterized by antibodies ("thyroid-stimulating immunoglobulins") which bind to the TSH-receptor, resulting in hyperthyroidism.

  - Clinical findings include the presence of a diffuse goiter, signs of hyperthyroidism (tachycardia, tremor, arrhythmia), and, in a minority, signs of ophthalmopathy.
  - Thyroid eye disease and pretibial myxedema differentiate Graves' disease from other causes of hyperthyroidism.

- *Toxic multinodular goiter* occurs typically in elderly subjects with a long-standing multinodular goiter (Plummer's disease).
- Occasionally solitary thyroid nodules can function autonomously leading to *toxic thyroid adenomas*.

Inflammatory Goiter

- *Hashimoto's disease* (chronic lymphocytic thyroiditis) is an organ-specific autoimmune disorder characterized by circulating antibodies directed against the thyroid peroxidase (TPO) or thyroglobulin (Tg) antigens. It is most common in middle-aged women.

  - Hashimoto's thyroiditis may after many years progress to hypothyroidism and FNABs are characterized by lymphocytic infiltration and associated Hürthle cell metaplasia.
  - Thyroid lymphoma may very rarely develop in goiters affected by Hashimoto's thyroiditis.

- *De Quervain's thyroiditis* is an inflammation of the thyroid, presumed secondary to a viral infection, that is associated with severe neck pain dramatically responsive to steroids.

  - Usually self-limiting over weeks and managed symptomatically.

- *Postpartum thyroiditis* is a self-limiting subacute inflammation of the thyroid gland which affects approximately 10 % of pregnancies and may be recurrent with each pregnancy.

  - This results in permanent hypothyroidism in around 50 % of affected women.

- *Riedel's struma or invasive fibrous thyroiditis* is rare and associated with a painless stony hard irregular gland that can mimic an anaplastic cancer.

  - The cause is unknown, but it may be associated with other similar inflammatory sclerosing conditions such as retroperitoneal fibrosis or fibrous mediastinitis.

Developmental Conditions

- *Thyroglossal duct cysts* are the most common upper neck midline lesions.

  - They are due to persistence of the stalk of epithelial cells that descend down from the floor of the primitive pharynx during development of the thyroid. The stalk normally undergoes atrophy at 6 weeks, but its persistence leads to cyst formation.
  - The mass moves on swallowing and/or protrusion of the tongue.
  - A fistula can result from spontaneous drainage of an infected cyst or from attempted drainage of a misdiagnosed neck abscess.

- *Ectopic thyroid* (*lingual thyroid*) is due to failure or abnormal descent of the thyroid during development.

  - Ninety percent of ectopic thyroid issue is associated with the dorsum of the tongue (Winslow and Weisberger 1997).
  - Usually asymptomatic but rarely may cause airway obstruction or dysphagia.
  - Associated with hypothyroidism in about 70 % of cases.

Assessment of Thyroid Enlargement

- As described in the chapter of evaluation of goiter, thyroid enlargement requires investigation in the form of clinical evaluation, laboratory tests to rule out thyroid dysfunction, and imaging with ultrasound and other modalities (especially if there are compressive symptoms). FNAB is performed in most nodular goitrous conditions.
- Although traditionally it was believed that a solitary thyroid nodule had a higher likelihood of malignancy, recent evidence indicates that the nodules in a multinodular goiter may harbor a similar risk of malignancy to that seen with clinically "solitary" nodules (Cooper et al. 2009).
- Current guidelines recommend FNA of the dominant nodule in MNG. In the presence of two or more nodules of >1 cm diameter, those with a suspicious appearance on ultrasound should be aspirated preferentially (Cooper et al. 2009).
- If a presumptive thyroglossal cyst is suprahyoid, a radioiodine or technetium scan may be helpful in excluding ectopic thyroid tissue.

Management

- Most euthyroid benign thyroid lesions do not require active management.
- British Thyroid Association (BTA) guidelines recommend repeat ultrasound-guided FNA after 6 months in patients with benign cytology (Thy2), following

which the patient can be discharged if benign cytology is confirmed (British Thyroid Association and Royal College of Physicians 2007).

- In some centers, particularly in the USA, patients are followed up at regular intervals, and any significant increase in size (more than 50 % change in volume or >20 % increase in at least two nodule dimensions) would warrant a repeat FNA and/or consideration for surgery (Cooper et al. 2009).

Indications for Surgery

- *Compression*: Patients presenting with features of tracheal or esophageal compression or venous outflow obstruction.
- *Suspicion of Malignancy*: Clinical or radiological evidence suspicious for malignancy, such as rapid growth, microcalcifications, irregular margins, or increased intra-nodular blood flow, may warrant surgery.
- *Cytological findings* suggestive or diagnostic of malignancy (Thy 3, 4, and 5) according to BTA guidelines (British Thyroid Association and Royal College of Physicians 2007).
- *Cosmetic Issues/Patient Preference*: This is controversial in view of the potential complications of surgery but may rarely be performed after obtaining an informed consent from the patient regarding the potential risks of hypocalcemia and hoarseness.
- *Hyperthyroidism*: In patients not responding to or intolerant of antithyroid drugs or who are unsuitable for radioiodine therapy (see Chap. 19)

Extent of Surgery

- *Hemithyroidectomy (lobectomy + isthmectomy)* is preferred in patients with unilateral nodular goiter, toxic adenoma, and unilateral cyst as well as in those undergoing diagnostic hemithyroidectomy for cytology suggestive of follicular neoplasm (Thy3).
- Subtotal thyroidectomy, which was formerly the preferred type of surgery, has fallen out of favor because of (1) a high chance of recurrence, (2) a higher rate of complication if revision surgery becomes necessary, and (3) a lack of functional benefit in preserving a small amount of thyroid tissue.
- *Near-total/total thyroidectomy* is the procedure of choice in patients with bilateral multinodular goiter. Patients with thyrotoxicosis require total thyroidectomy.
- Surgical procedure for thyroglossal cyst is the *Sistrunk* procedure which involves removal of the duct tract along with the body of the hyoid between the lesser horns and a core of muscle up to the foramen cecum.
- Lingual thyroid, if symptomatic, can be excised by a *transhyoid/lateral pharyngotomy* or by *transoral laser excision*.

Nonsurgical Treatments

- *Administration of Radioactive Iodine 131*

- The role of radioiodine therapy in toxic goiter has been well described (Royal College of Physicians. Radioiodine in the management of benign thyroid disease: Clinical guidelines. Report of a Working Party. London: RCP 2007).
- A number of studies have indicated that radioiodine may reduce thyroid volume in patients with nontoxic multinodular goiter, with size reductions ranging from 40 to 60 % within 1–2 years of ^{131}I therapy (Hegedus et al. 2003).
- Disadvantages include:

   - Acute worsening of compressive symptoms during therapy
   - Slow variable response
   - Small long-term risk of cancer induction outside the thyroid bed with large doses which are required for large goiters (Huysmans et al. 1996)

- This approach is therefore usually limited to older patients who are unfit for surgery.

- *Administration of Suppressive Doses of Levothyroxine*

   - This approach is based on the hypothesis that TSH suppression caused by high oral doses of levothyroxine will decrease goiter size (Berghout et al. 1990).
   - Not currently recommended because of variable response (only 25 % of nodules shrink more than 50 %) and concerns about systemic effects of long-term serum TSH suppression on bone and the cardiovascular system leading to osteoporosis and atrial fibrillation respectively (Cooper and Biondi 2012).

- Benign Thyroid Disease in Children

   - Nodular goiter is uncommon in children. Most goiters in children are physiological and may present as diffuse enlargements during puberty. Developmental conditions, such as thyroglossal duct cysts, are more common in children.
   - Diagnostic work-up and management of these lesions are the same as in adults.
   - Solitary thyroid nodule when seen in children should be viewed with a high index of suspicion, since there is a higher incidence of malignancy than in adults (16–25 %).

Pearls and Pitfalls
Pearls

- Most benign thyroid diseases do not require surgical management
- Total thyroidectomy is the procedure of choice for patients with thyrotoxicosis and requires close monitoring by the endocrinologist during the perioperative period
- Thyroid nodules in children, although rare, have a higher risk of malignancy than in adults

Pitfalls

- Thyroid surgery is occasionally performed for benign thyroid diseases without definite indication
- Subtotal thyroidectomy is no longer advised for toxic/bilateral nodular goiter
- Treating multinodular goiter with TSH suppression by thyroxine is not recommended

References

Berghout A, Wiersinga WM, et al. Comparison of placebo with L-thyroxine or with carbimazole for treatment of sporadic non-toxic goitre. Lancet. 1990;336:193–7.

British Thyroid Association and Royal College of Physicians. 2007. Guidelines for the management of thyroid cancer. www.british-thyroid-association.org.

Cooper DS, Biondi B. Subclinical thyroid disease. Lancet. 2012;379(9821):1142–54.

Cooper DS, Doherty GM, Haugen BR, et al. Revised American Thyroid Association Management Guidelines for patients with thyroid nodules and differentiated thyroid cancer. Thyroid. 2009; 19(11):1167–214.

Hegedus L, Bonnema SJ, Bennedbaek FN. Management of simple nodular goitre: current status and future perspectives. Endocr Rev. 2003;24(1):102–32.

Huysmans DA, Buijs WC, Vande Ven MT, et al. Dosimetry and risk estimates of radioiodine therapy for large multinodular goitres. J Nucl Med. 1996;37:2072–9.

Matovinevic J. Endemic goitre and cretinism at the dawn of the 3rd millennium. Annu Rev Nutr. 1983;3:341–2.

Royal College of Physicians. Radioiodine in the management of benign thyroid disease: Clinical guidelines. Report of a Working Party. London: RCP; 2007.

Winslow CP, Weisberger EC. Lingual thyroid and neoplastic change: a review of the literature and description of a case. Otolaryngol Head Neck Surg. 1997;117:S100.

Chapter 14
Management of the Indeterminate Thyroid Nodule

Dae Kim and Jeremy Freeman

Introduction

Thyroid nodules are very common. Although palpable nodules in the thyroid gland are present in only 4–7 %, as many as 67 % of the population are detectable by ultrasound (Gharib and Goellner 1993).

Initial evaluation of thyroid nodules using US-guided FNAC is now well established, and since its introduction in the 1970s, its routine use has decreased the number of patients requiring surgery and has increased the yield of thyroid malignancy in those patients who undergo surgery (Cooper et al. 2006). Large-scale experiences published report FNAC diagnoses of approximately 60–70 % benign, 5 % malignant, 5–15 % non-diagnostic, and 15–25 % indeterminate (Gharib and Goellner 1993).

The management of patients with indeterminate or suspicious FNA specimens (up to 30 % of FNAs in some studies) still remains problematic, and most of these patients go on to diagnostic surgical resection. Given that 12–50 % of these are histologically proven to be malignant, up to 88 % of patients may undergo unnecessary surgery (Banks et al. 2008). Further, the optimal operation recommended (total thyroidectomy versus lobectomy) is dependent upon whether the nodule is benign or malignant, a fact not available until after surgery. Many patients may require a second completion surgery.

The overall management of thyroid nodules and the threshold for (and rate of) diagnostic surgery for suspicious and indeterminate nodules vary significantly as a

D. Kim (✉)
Department of Otolaryngology, Head and Neck Surgery, Queen Alexandra Hospital, Portsmouth, UK
e-mail: daekim72@yahoo.co.uk

J. Freeman
Department of Otolaryngology, Head and Neck Surgery,
Mount Sinai Hospital, Toronto, Canada

J.C. Watkinson, D.M. Scott-Coombes (eds.), *Tips and Tricks in Endocrine Surgery*, 123
DOI 10.1007/978-1-4471-2146-6_14, © Springer-Verlag London 2014

result of differing cultural attitudes to malignancy risk (pro-surgery in North America and the Far East compared to Europe).

The advent of alternative surgical techniques such as minimally invasive thyroidectomy (e.g., MIVAT) and robot-assisted "scarless-in-neck" thyroidectomy may affect the rate of diagnostic surgery in centers/regions that offer these alternative surgical options.

Definition of an "Indeterminate Nodule": Thy/Bethesda Classifications

It is important to define clearly what we mean by an indeterminate thyroid nodule. Traditionally thyroid FNA cytology specimens have been classified into three broad diagnostic categories: benign, malignant, or indeterminate. However, it was quickly realized that the indeterminate category was too broad.

Indeterminate thyroid FNA cytology encompasses a cohort of microscopic findings that suggest concern for the possibility of a thyroid malignancy, yet are inconclusive. Descriptions range from indeterminate, to atypical cellularity, to suspicious for a follicular neoplasm or even suggestive of malignancy; all conferring similar malignancy risk. Consensus terminology for classifying indeterminate FNA cytology specimens has been lacking for many years. This is evident from the widely variable rate of indeterminate thyroid FNAC results in the medical literature (Cibas and Sanchez 2008). This is also partly due to the intraobserver and interobserver variation in the cytologic characteristics that are reported as indeterminate.

In an attempt to address these problems, several stratified classification systems have been proposed aimed at standardizing cytology nomenclature and improving consistency in reporting. Both the British Thyroid Association and the American Thyroid Association have introduced or endorsed their respective FNAC reporting systems (commonly referred to as the "Thy classification" and the Bethesda classification) (Table 14.1).

The US National Cancer Institute-sponsored Thyroid State of Science conference in Bethesda (2007) standardized the morphological criteria and diagnostic terminology for the reporting of thyroid FNAC. A six-tiered diagnostic classification was proposed: "The Bethesda System for Reporting Thyroid Cytopathology (TBSRTC)" (Cibas and Ali 2009). A major feature of the new system was the creation of an additional category designated: atypia of undetermined significance (AUS)/follicular lesion of undetermined significance (FLUS). The system currently in most widespread use in the UK is the joint British Thyroid Association/Royal College of Physicians Thy1-5 classification, although first produced in 2002 (British Thyroid Association RCoP 2007). More recently, the Royal College of Pathologists produced a modified version in 2009, which, in parallel with the US Bethesda System, also described six subcategories that are very much similar in both description and categorization (Cross et al. 2009). Both systems not only facilitate interinstitutional communication by standardizing cytology language but also facilitate

Table 14.1 The RCPath-modified BTA nomenclature and comparison with the US Bethesda System for Reporting Thyroid Cytopathology

Royal College of Pathologists-modified BTA nomenclature	US Bethesda System (BSRTC)	Risk of malignancy (%)
Thy1: Nondiagnostic	I: Nondiagnostic	0–10
	Virtually acellular specimen	
	Other (blood, clotting artifacts, etc.)	
Thy1c: Nondiagnostic – cystic lesion	Cyst fluid only	
Thy2: Nonneoplastic	II: Benign	0–3
	Consistent with a benign follicular nodule or lymphocytic thyroiditis or granulomatous (subacute) thyroiditis	
Thy2c: Nonneoplastic, cystic lesion		
Thy3a: Neoplasm possible – atypia	III: Atypia of undetermined significance (AUS) or follicular lesion of undetermined significance (FLUS)	5–15
Thy3f: Neoplasm possible – suggestive of follicular neoplasm	IV: Follicular neoplasm or suspicious for follicular neoplasm	15–30
	Specify if Hürthle cell (oncocytic) type	
Thy4: Suspicious of malignancy	V: Suspicious for malignancy	60–75
	Suspicious for papillary/medullary/metastatic/lymphoma	
	Carcinoma	
Thy5: Malignant	VI: Malignant	97–100

decision-making process by providing a set of diagnostic categories each with an associated malignancy risk and recommendation for clinical management decision.

It is important to point out that the associated risk figures quoted in these classification systems are "average" values, and several individual institutions have since their introduction have audited their performance figures, and some have shown their risk figures for each diagnostic category to significantly differ from the "typical" values proposed in the USA and UK classification systems (Broome and Solorzano 2011; Yehuda et al. 2007; MSH). Each institution should therefore audit their own FNAC "performance" and associated risk of malignancy against the "standard" quoted values and use them when consenting their individual patient population.

Risk Factors of Malignancy

Although FNAC of thyroid nodules represent the most sensitive and specific test for malignancy, additional assessment of other risk factors would further improve the diagnostic rate of thyroid nodules. Efforts to further improve the management of these patients with indeterminate FNAC results have focused on identifying clinical, sonographic, and more recently molecular characteristics that predict malignancy.

Clinical Risk Factors

Clinical variables have been investigated for a long time with regard to their ability to predict malignancy. High-risk history/examination features such as hoarseness, fixation of thyroid nodule to adjacent structures, nodal disease, strong family history or genetic conditions (e.g., medullary thyroid carcinoma, Cowden's syndrome), and prior radiation exposure are well known but are relatively uncommon findings. Other major clinical factors that have been investigated are age, gender, and tumor size (Fiore et al. 2009):

Age: Generally high risk if less than 20 or older than 70.

Gender: Although females are 2–3 times more likely to suffer a thyroid cancer, nodule in a male is associated with 1.5–2-fold increased risk compared with a female.

Tumor size: This feature is the least consistently found to be a risk factor determinator. Some studies have shown tumors larger than 3–4 cm more likely to be malignant.

Serum TSH: Significantly higher levels of TSH are present in patients who are subsequently diagnosed with thyroid cancer, suggesting it could be used as an adjunct to FNAC (Fiore et al. 2009).

Sonographic Risk Factors

There have been advances in associating sonographic features of thyroid nodules to malignancy risk. Hypoechogenicity, solid composition, microcalcifications, irregular or ill-defined margins, an absent sonolucent rim (or "halo"), and Doppler evidence of increased blood flow in the center of the nodule are associated with an increased risk of malignancy (Alexander 2008). True microcalcification appears to be the highest predictor of malignancy. Of course associated abnormal lymph nodes are highly suspicious for a primary thyroid malignancy.

Molecular Risk Factors

Much effort has been made to identify molecular markers of thyroid malignancy. The most widely studied and most promising markers are BRAF, RAS, PAX8-PPAR-g, Galectin-3, and RET-PTC rearrangements. Recent research has shown in particular, *BRAF* mutational analysis to enhance diagnostic accuracy when used in conjunction with FNAC (Nikiforov and Nikiforova 2011). Several large centers in the USA now routinely test all thyroid FNAC samples for *BRAF* mutation as positivity provides both diagnostic and prognostic information. Further, in the USA (and perhaps shortly in Europe), there is increasing use of the commercial "genetic" testing Afirma (Veracyte Inc: http://www.veracyte.com/afirma/) on indeterminate FNAC samples that appears to be very accurate. This panel of tests is presently very expensive but with eventual drop in costs its use may become widespread and points towards the expected future of molecular/gene testing in routine clinical practice.

Recent Advances in Thyroid Nodule Diagnosis

Contrast-Enhanced "Microbubble" US

Nanoparticles have been used to enhance both the functional and structural information from US scans of thyroid nodules, and these show early promise. In particular, use of microbubbles of air encased in lipid layer has been shown to provide more sensitive detection of tumor micro-deposits and the associated early alterations to vascularity within both thyroid nodules and lymph nodes (Nemec et al. 2012).

US Elastography

This technique estimates tissue stiffness by measuring the degree of tissue's deformation in response to external force. Early studies have shown real promise in accurately predicting malignancy in solid nodules (Rago et al. 2007). It is less effective in partly/cystic lesions and in multinodular goiters where multiple nodules coincide.

CT-PET

Early studies suggest avidity for FGD to be associated with increased risk for thyroid cancer (Mitchell et al. 2005). However, routine use is precluded by the radiation exposure and prohibitive costs.

Core Biopsy

Recent research has suggested US-guided core biopsy of thyroid nodules to provide greater diagnostic accuracy than repeat FNA in those with nondiagnostic or indeterminate nodule (Na et al. 2012).

Pearls

- Up to 25 % of thyroid FNACs are indeterminate and remain a common management/diagnostic dilemma.
- The rate of indeterminate FNAC rate varies from institution to institution. It is important in defining what an indeterminate thyroid nodule represents at each institution is important.
- Importance of agreeing and defining the thyroid FNAC classification system at your institution.
- Your own unit's thyroid FNAC performance figures should be audited and compared.
- Combining FNAC with a multimodality risk assessment, including clinical risk scoring, sonographic features, and molecular markers will guide the optimal surgical decision-making and help to reduce unnecessary surgery rates.
- Molecular/genetic testing of indeterminate thyroid nodules to enhance present diagnostic tests should be explored further, and indeed commercial testing may be widely employed in the near future.
- Other newer diagnostic modalities such as core biopsy, elastography, and microbubble US may prove to be valuable in the near future but require further clinical research.

References

Alexander EKJ. Approach to the patient with a cytologically indeterminate thyroid nodule. Clin Endocrinol Metab. 2008;93(11):4175–82.

Banks ND, Kowalski J, Tsai H, Somerveil H, Tufano R, Dackiw APB, Marohn MR, Clark DP, Umbricht CB, Zeiger MA. A diagnostic predictor model for indeterminate or suspicious thyroid FNA samples. Thyroid. 2008;18(9):933–41.

British Thyroid Association RCoP. Guidelines for the management of thyroid cancer. 2nd ed. Report of the Thyroid Cancer Guidelines Update Group. London: RCP; 2007. www.rcplondon. ac.uk/pubs/contents/5e0be7d7-0726-48af-a510-5cc5b9ec57d.pdf.

Broome JT, Solorzano CC. The Impact of atypia/follicular lesion of undetermined significance on the rate of malignancy in thyroid fine-needle aspiration: Evaluation of the Bethesda System for Reporting Thyroid Cytopathology. Surgery. 2011;150:1234–41.

Cibas ES, Ali SZ. The Bethesda system for reporting thyroid cytopathology. Thyroid. 2009;19:1159–65.

Cibas ES, Sanchez MA. The National Cancer Institute thyroid fine-needle aspiration state-of-the-science conference: inspiration for a uniform terminology linked to management guidelines. Cancer Cytopathol. 2008;114:71–3.

Cooper DS, Doherty GM, Haugen BR, Kloos RT, Lee SL, Mandel SJ, Mazzaferri EL, McIver B, Sherman SL, Tuttle RM. Management guidelines for patients with thyroid nodules and differentiated thyroid cancer. Thyroid. 2006;16:1–33.

Cross P, Chandra A, Giles T, Johnson S, Kocjan G, Poller D, Stephenson T. Guidance on the reporting of thyroid cytology specimens. Nov 2009. www.rcpath.org.

Fiore E, Rago T, Provenzale MA, Scutari M, Ugolini C, Basolo F, Di Coscio G, Berti P, Grasso L, Elisei R, Pinchera A, Vitti P. Lower levels of TSH are associated with a lower risk of papillary thyroid cancer in patients with thyroid nodular disease: thyroid autonomy may play a protective role. Endocr Relat Cancer. 2009;16(4):1251–60.

Gharib H, Goellner JR. Fine-needle aspiration biopsy of the thyroid: an appraisal. Ann Intern Med. 1993;118:282–9.

Mitchell JC, Grant F, Evenson AR, Parker JA, Hasselgren PO, Parangi S. Preoperative evaluation of thyroid nodules with 18FDG-PET/CT. Surgery. 2005;138:1166–75.

Na DG, Kim JH, Sung JY, Baek JH, Jung KC, Lee H, Yoo H. Core-needle biopsy is more useful than repeat fine-needle aspiration in thyroid nodules read as nondiagnostic or atypia of undetermined significance by the Bethesda system for reporting thyroid cytopathology. Thyroid. 2012;22(5):468–75.

Nemec U, Nemec SF, Novotny C, Weber M, Czemy C, Krestan CR. Quantitative evaluation of contrast enhances ultrasound after intravenous administration of a microbubble contrast agent for differentiation of benign and malignant thyroid nodules: assessment of diagnostic accuracy. Eur Radiol. 2012;22(6):1357–65.

Nikiforov YE, Nikiforova MN. Molecular genetics and diagnosis of thyroid cancer. Nat Rev Endocrinol. 2011;7:569–80.

Rago T, Santini F, Scutari M, Pinchera A, Vitt P. Elastography: new developments in ultrasound for predicting malignancy in thyroid nodules. J Clin Endocrinol Metab. 2007;92:2917–22.

Yehuda M, Payne RJ, Seaberg RM, MacMillan C, Freeman JL. Fine-needle aspiration biopsy of the thyroid: atypical cytopathological features. Arch Otolaryngol Head Neck Surg. 2007;133:477–80.

Chapter 15
Differentiated Thyroid Cancer

Osama Al Hamarneh and John C. Watkinson

Background

- Thyroid cancer is rare, making around 1 % of all cancers.
- Evidence suggests an increasing incidence, with an estimated 33,600 new cases in 2008 in the EU countries and 37,000 new cases in the USA in 2009. Survival rates remain otherwise static.
- Types of DTC include papillary (85 %) and follicular (15 %), all arising from thyroid follicular cells.
- Accurate diagnosis, treatment, and long-term follow-up through a multidisciplinary approach are essential to achieve and maintain survival rates.
- High-risk patients include males, age >5 years or <14 years, solitary thyroid nodule, tumor >4 cm, family history, history of irradiation, extracapsular disease, and extrathyroidal disease.
- Several oncogenes have been shown to play an important role in thyroid carcinogenesis and development.

Presentation

- The commonest presentation is by far a solitary thyroid nodule, which carries a 10 % risk of malignancy.

O. Al Hamarneh, MBBS, MRCS, DOHNS, MD (✉)
ENT Department, Queen Elizabeth Hospital, Mindelsohn Way,
Edgbaston, Birmingham, West Midlands B15 2WB, UK
e-mail: ohamarneh@gmail.com

J.C. Watkinson
ENT Department, Queen Elizabeth Hospital, Birmingham, UK

J.C. Watkinson, D.M. Scott-Coombes (eds.), *Tips and Tricks in Endocrine Surgery*,
DOI 10.1007/978-1-4471-2146-6_15, © Springer-Verlag London 2014

- Other presentations include voice changes/stridor associated with a thyroid nodule/ goiter, thyroid nodule during pregnancy, cervical lymphadenopathy associated with a thyroid nodule, and/or rapidly enlarging painless goiter over a period of weeks.
- Pediatric thyroid nodules are four times more likely to carry a diagnosis of thyroid cancer than adult nodules.
- Only 50 % of children with DTC present with a solitary thyroid nodule. In 40–60 % of patients, a painless noninflammatory metastatic cervical mass is the presenting symptom.
- Children commonly present with advanced disease. At presentation, 70 % of patients have extensive regional nodal involvement, and 10–20 % of patients have distant metastasis.

Assessment (See Also Chap. 12)

History and Examination

- Ascertain family history and irradiation therapy, particularly in childhood.
- PTC nodules tend to be harder than FTC nodules and have a higher rate of nodal metastasis.
- When examining the neck, maintain a high degree of suspicion, as lymph node metastasis can be difficult to palpate.
- Always perform direct fiberoptic endoscopy to assess the vocal cords for any paralysis or tumor invasion.

Investigations

- Blood tests should include TSH, T3, T4, thyroid antibodies, and calcium levels.
- Elevated TSH is associated with an increased risk of malignancy.
- FNAC should be done preferably under USS guidance. USS provides the added benefit of identifying suspicious nodes and may alter surgical approach.
- Excisional biopsy under general anesthesia is recommended in children younger than 10 as FNAC is often not practical.
- MRI or CT scans (*without the use of iodinated contrast*) should be performed in cases with suspected retrosternal extension, fixed tumors (local invasion ± vocal cord paralysis), and when hemoptysis is reported.

Staging

- All patients should be staged by clinical and pathological TNM staging (Tables 15.1 and 15.2).
- Other staging systems include AMES, DAMES, and MACIS, however not widely used.

Table 15.1 TNM staging for thyroid carcinoma

Stage	
TX	Primary tumor cannot be assessed
T0	No evidence of primary tumor
T1a	Tumor 1 cm or less in greatest dimension, limited to the thyroid
T1b	Tumor 1–2 cm in greatest dimension, limited to the thyroid
T2	Tumor more than 2 cm but not more than 4 cm in greatest dimension, limited to the thyroid
T3	Tumor more than 4 cm in greatest dimension, limited to the thyroid or any tumor with minimal extrathyroid extension (e.g., extension to sternothyroid muscle or perithyroid soft tissues)
T4a	Tumor of any size extending beyond the thyroid capsule and invades any of the following: subcutaneous soft tissues, larynx, trachea, esophagus, recurrent laryngeal nerve
T4b	Tumor invades prevertebral fascia, mediastinal vessels, or encases carotid artery
NX	Regional lymph nodes cannot be assessed
N0	No regional lymph node metastasis
N1	Regional lymph node metastasis
N1a	Metastasis in level VI (pretracheal and paratracheal, including prelaryngeal and Delphian lymph nodes)
N1b	Metastasis in other unilateral, bilateral, or contralateral cervical or upper/superior mediastinal lymph nodes
cM0	Clinically no distant metastasis
cM1	Distant metastasis clinically
pTNM	Pathological classification
pN0	Histological examination of a selective neck dissection specimen will ordinarily include six or more lymph nodes. If the lymph nodes are negative, but the number ordinarily examined is not met, classify as pN0
pM1	Distant metastasis proven microscopically

Used with the permission of the American Joint Committee on Cancer (AJCC), Chicago, Illinois. The original source for this material is the *AJCC Cancer Staging Manual*, Seventh Edition (2010) published by Springer Science and Business Media LLC, www.springer.com

Table 15.2 Stage grouping for papillary and follicular carcinoma

Papillary and follicular thyroid cancer (age <45 years):			
Stage	**T**	**N**	**M**
I	Any T	Any N	M0
II	Any T	Any N	M1
Papillary and follicular; differentiated (age ≥45 years):			
Stage	**T**	**N**	**M**
I	T1	N0	M0
II	T2	N0	M0
III	T3	N0	M0
IVA	T1-3	N1a	M0
	T4a	N1b	M0
IVB	T4b	Any N	M0
IVC	Any T	Any N	M1

Used with the permission of the American Joint Committee on Cancer (AJCC), Chicago, Illinois. The original source for this material is the *AJCC Cancer Staging Manual*, Seventh Edition (2010) published by Springer Science and Business Media LLC, www.springer.com

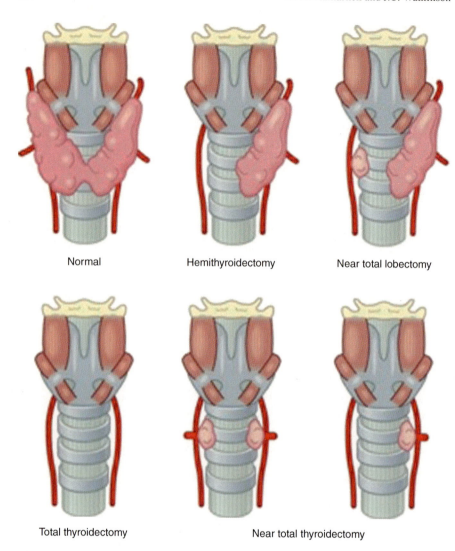

Fig. 15.1 Surgical options for the management of DTC (Reproduced with permission from Watkinson JC, Gilbert RW, Arnold H, editors. Stell and Maran's textbook of head and neck surgery and oncology. 5th ed. London: Hodder Arnold; 2012. p. 433, Fig 23.12)

Prognostic Factors

- Uncontrolled prognostic factors that are considered poor include age >45, males, tumor size (Fig. 15.1), tumor grade, tall cell variant of PTC, FTC with extensive vascular invasion, local invasion or distant metastasis, and nodal metastasis especially in elderly patients.

- Controlled prognostic factors include the extent of surgery, experience of surgeon, treatment with postoperative radioiodine, and any delays in therapy.
- The 10-year overall relative survival rates for patients in the USA are 93 % for PTC and 85 % for FTC.

Treatment of DTC

- The mainstay of treatment is surgery with radioactive iodine remnant ablation and thyroxine suppression through a multidisciplinary team.
- Debate still exists regarding the optimal operation for DTC, particularly in low-risk disease. Surgical options are summarized in Figure 1.
- Lobectomy/hemithyroidectomy should include the isthmus in all patients. Completion surgery, when indicated, is recommended within 8 weeks of histological diagnosis.
- Total thyroidectomy is indicated in patients with indeterminate nodules who have large tumors (>4 cm), when marked atypia is seen on biopsy, when the biopsy reading is "suspicious for papillary carcinoma," in patients with a family history of thyroid carcinoma and in patients with a history of radiation exposure.
- Prophylactic central compartment neck dissection should be done for all tumors over 1 cm in high-risk patients.
- While lobectomy might be considered for stages I and II DTC, albeit a 5–10 % risk of recurrence, total thyroidectomy with or without neck dissection is the standard treatment option for stage III.
- Surgery for stage IV DTC should include excising symptomatic metastasis.
- In pregnant women, the optimal time of surgery is still debatable with recommendations to perform surgery either at the second trimester or after delivery.
- In children, especially under 10, DTC should be treated aggressively; however, they carry a much better prognosis than adult DTC.

Surgical Management of PTC

- PTC can be multifocal in up to 80 % of cases and that 50 % of foci can be in the contralateral lobe. Despite this, local recurrence rates of PTC are only 5 %.
- Frozen section histology may be of use is suspected PTC (Thy4).
- Tumors <1 cm with no other clinical features can be adequately treated by lobectomy and thyroxine suppression therapy.
- Total or near-total thyroidectomy is indicated for tumors >1 cm, multifocal disease, familial disease, history of irradiation, extrathyroidal extension, lymph nodes involvement, or distant metastasis.

Surgical Management of FTC

- Thy 3 cytology mandates at least a diagnostic hemithyroidectomy. Frozen section is not recommended in suspected FTC.
- A diagnosis of minimally invasive FTC without vascular invasion, <2 cm in a low-risk patient, can be managed by a lobectomy and thyroxine suppression therapy following MDT discussion and informed consent.
- Cases of low-risk minimally invasive FTC between 2 and 4 cm should be discussed individually at MDT.
- All other cases should be offered a total or near-total thyroidectomy.
- Hürthle cell (follicular oncocytic), a variant of FTC, tends to be a more aggressive tumor and should be treated with total (completion) thyroidectomy.
- In children, benign tumors such as follicular adenomas should be considered at risk for tumor progression toward FTC, and they must be surgically treated.

Pearls and Pitfalls
Pearls

- The most common presentation of DTC is a solitary thyroid nodule in a euthyroid patient
- Thy3 necessitate at least a diagnostic lobectomy including the isthmus
- Some cases can be treated with lobectomy and TSH suppression after informed consent
- Follow-up is lifelong with clinical assessment, serum Tg, and TSH suppression

Pitfalls

- Avoid treating patients outside a thyroid MDT
- Failure to evaluate the vocal cords prior to surgery
- Avoid iodinated contrast when requesting a CT scan
- Do not delay completion surgery more than 8 weeks' post-histology outcome

---

Recommended Reading

American Thyroid Association (ATA) Guidelines Taskforce on Thyroid Nodules and Differentiated Thyroid Cancer, Cooper DS, Doherty GM, Haugen BR, Kloos RT, Lee SL, Mandel SJ, Mazzaferri EL, McIver B, Pacini F, Schlumberger M, Sherman SI, Steward DL, Tuttle RM. Revised American thyroid association management guidelines for patients with thyroid nodules and differentiated thyroid cancer. Thyroid. 2009;19:1167–214.

British Thyroid Association and Royal College of Physicians. Guidelines for the management of thyroid cancer. In: Perros P, editor. Report of the Thyroid Cancer Guidelines Update Group. London: Royal College of Physicians; 2007.

Roland NJ, Paleri V, editors. Head and neck cancer: multidisciplinary management guidelines. 4th ed. London: ENT UK; 2011.

Chapter 16
Medullary Thyroid Cancer

Barney Harrison and Bruno Carnaille

Definition

Medullary thyroid cancer (MTC) arises from C cells of neural crest origin. C cells are found in the middle and upper third of the thyroid, adjacent to thyroid follicles, and produce calcitonin. The physiological role of calcitonin is unclear and despite markedly increased levels in the circulation in patients with advanced MTC, it has no apparent clinical effect. Other peptides released by MTC include CEA and those responsible for systemic symptoms (diarrhea, flushing) in patients with widespread disease. An increase in C cell numbers (C cell hyperplasia) is found as a precursor of MTC in MEN 2 kindred but may be found in patients with hypercalcemia, thyroiditis, and follicular tumors and male, obese smokers.

Incidence

MTC accounts for approximately 3–5 % of thyroid cancers with maximum incidence in 70–75-year-olds (4.4 per million per year); the estimated incidence in the UK is up to 25 new cases per year. MTC prevalence in patients with nodular thyroid disease who are screened with basal calcitonin levels is reported as 0.4–1.8 %. The rarity of this disease mandates that patients, and when appropriate are their families, are treated by a multidisciplinary team in the Cancer Center.

B. Harrison, MBBS, MS, FRCS Eng (✉)
Department of Endocrine Surgery, Royal Hallamshire Hospital,
Glossop Road, Sheffield S10 2JF, UK
e-mail: barney.harrison@sth.nhs.uk

B. Carnaille, MD
Department of Endocrine Surgery, University Hospital, Hopital Huriez, Lille 59037, France
e-mail: bruno.carnaille@chru-lille.fr

J.C. Watkinson, D.M. Scott-Coombes (eds.), *Tips and Tricks in Endocrine Surgery*,
DOI 10.1007/978-1-4471-2146-6_16, © Springer-Verlag London 2014

Approximately 25 % of MTC cases are genetically determined caused by germ-line mutations in the *RET* proto-oncogene (chromosome 10) that result in multiple endocrine neoplasia (MEN) 2A (85 %), MEN 2B (5 %), and familial MTC (5–15 %). The syndromes are inherited in an autosomal dominant manner with age-related penetrance and variable expression; MTC is expressed in almost all gene carriers.

Clinical Features

Sporadic MTC typically presents in the 4th and 5th decade; the sex ratio is equal. A thyroid mass is the presenting complaint in at least 75 %, with cervical node enlargement in 40–50 % of patients. Diarrhea, flushing, and bone pain are reported in 20–30 %, and approximately 20 % of patients will have evidence of metastases in the liver, lungs, and bones.

In genetically determined disease, MEN 2B will often present in the first and second decade, MEN 2A in the second and third decade, and FMTC in the fourth and fifth decade. Pheochromocytoma (unilateral or bilateral) will occur in as many as 55 % of MEN 2 patients; annual screening should start from the age of 10 in patients with RET mutations in codons 918, 634, and 630 and from the age of 20 in the remainder. Hyperparathyroidism occurs in up to one third of patients with MEN 2A. Patients with FMTC have none of the extrathyroidal manifestations seen in MEN 2, and it requires multiple members of the same kindred with this phenotype to determine a clear diagnosis. MEN 2B is associated with very early onset and metastatic potential, de novo mutation in 50 % and a typical phenotype that becomes more overt with increasing age (Table 16.1).

Diagnosis and Investigations

FNA of a thyroid or lymph node mass will typically identify oval- or spindle-shaped cells with pleomorphic nuclei and eosinophilic cytoplasm. Immunohistochemistry will be positive for calcitonin and CEA. Core biopsy may in addition reveal malignant cells with a low mitotic rate and amyloid.

Table 16.1 Phenotype of MEN 2B

Medullary thyroid cancer (100 %)
Pheochromocytoma (50 %)
Multiple neuroma of lip, tongue, and buccal mucosa (>90 %)
Prominent corneal nerve fibers
Ganglioneuromatosis of the GI tract (producing constipation)
Marfanoid habitus
Dry eyes
Foot abnormalities
Hyperflexible joints

An elevated serum calcitonin confirms the diagnosis of MTC and should be measured in all patients prior to surgery as it is a good marker of disease extent (as is CEA). Distant metastasis can be found in patients with calcitonin of as low as 150–400 pg/mL. When there is uncertainty about the histological diagnosis or potential for false-positive calcitonin levels (autoimmune thyroid disease, hypercalcemia, foregut-derived neuroendocrine tumors, and renal failure), a pentagastrin/calcium stimulation test can be performed. Peak values of calcitonin occur at 1–2 min after intravenous pentagastrin/calcium injection.

Pheochromocytoma must be excluded in all patients on diagnosis of MTC by the measurement of urine metanephrines, normetanephrines, and fractionated catecholamine levels in a 24-h urine collection and/or by measurement of plasma normetanephrine/metanephrine levels which have high sensitivity for the detection of pheochromocytoma.

Serum calcium and if elevated PTH levels should be measured before operation because if elevated indicates hyperparathyroidism and the presence of familial disease.

All patients with MTC should be offered *RET* mutation analysis to identify those patients with genetically determined disease – even in patients with apparently sporadic disease, the prevalence of a germline *RET* mutation is more than 7 %.

Ultrasound scan of the neck can identify unsuspected multiple/bilateral thyroid nodules that give a clue that there is familial disease and assess lymph nodes for the presence of metastatic disease. CT or MRI of the neck and mediastinum will in some patients identify unsuspected extrathyroidal spread and lymph node metastases below the brachiocephalic vein inaccessible at neck surgery. The absence of metastatic foci on cross-sectional imaging of the liver and lungs does not exclude the presence of miliary tumor foci below the limit of scan resolution.

Laryngoscopy is indicated in all patients prior to surgery.

Surgery

The aim of neck surgery in patients with MTC is to obtain local control and provide the optimum chance of clinical and biochemical cure. Total thyroidectomy and central compartment lymph node dissection are the minimum interventions that should be performed when the diagnosis is made prior to surgery. If the diagnosis is made after thyroid lobectomy or total thyroidectomy, because lymph node metastases in level 6 occur so frequently (up to 80 % of patients), completion central compartment node dissection is mandated. The frequency of lateral compartment node metastases is high – ipsilateral 30–80 % and contralateral 19–50 % – so in patients without evidence of distant metastases, ipsilateral lateral compartment selective neck dissection (levels 2–5) should be also be performed. In patients with 2 or more lymph node compartments positive for metastases, cure is not achieved, so in the absence of radiological/palpable nodal disease in the contralateral lateral compartment, it is not unreasonable to delay further lateral neck until required on the basis of evident disease.

Tips for Surgery

- If you get it right the first time, you will reduce the need for reoperation in the central neck.
- Aim to preserve recurrent/superior laryngeal nerves and parathyroid glands.
- In patients with elevated basal calcitonin and or lymph node metastases, perform total thyroidectomy and central/and at least, ipsilaterallateral compartment selective neck dissection.
- In patients with infra-brachiocephalic lymph node involvement (or high risk on the basis of a T4 tumor), transsternal mediastinal node dissection should be performed or considered to minimize the risk of future airway/esophageal/recurrent laryngeal nerve compromise.
- In patients who present with distant metastases, survival may be prolonged. On that basis, total thyroidectomy and central compartment node dissection should be considered and, if required, resection of symptomatic disease in the lateral neck or mediastinum.
- If incidental sporadic micro-MTC (<1 cm) is found after hemithyroidectomy with normal postoperative basal and pentagastrin- /calcium-stimulated calcitonin, no further surgery is required.
- For all other sized MTC diagnosed after thyroid surgery when the basal calcitonin is normal but stimulated calcitonin is elevated, perform completion thyroidectomy and central neck lymph node dissection.
- The timing of risk reduction (prophylactic) surgery in *RET* gene-positive individuals is based not only on the codon affected but also on patient age and calcitonin level. Thyroidectomy is recommended at the following ages:

Highest risk carriers (codons 883, 918) within the first year of life
High-risk carriers (codons 609, 611, 618, 620, 630, 634) before the age of 5 years
Least high-risk carriers (codons 768, 790, 791, 804, 891) before the age of 10 years

- If the basal calcitonin is normal prior to risk reduction surgery and there are no clinical or radiological features to the contrary, lymphadenectomy can be avoided.

Outcomes

Approximately half of patients who present with palpable disease in the thyroid will develop locoregional recurrence. Patients with node-negative disease (pN0) after appropriate surgery are likely to be disease-free at 5 years. Survival rates (cause specific) for patients with MTC are variously reported as 69–97 % at 5 years and 56–96 % at 10 years. More than 50 % of patients with sporadic disease will die of MTC. Biochemical cure is associated with >95 % survival at 10 years. In the presence of systemic symptoms, a third of patients die within 5 years. Calcitonin doubling times after surgery of less than 12 months indicate a worse prognosis.

Detection and Treatment of Persistent/Recurrent Disease

In patients with persistent or recurrent high calcitonin/CEA levels, important considerations are:

- Was the surgery (particularly the extent of lymph node excision) less than that recommended or appropriate?
- Is the calcitonin elevation caused by disease in the neck or mediastinum and therefore amenable to surgery?
- Will further surgery result in cure, improved survival, or most effective local control?

Reoperation in selected patients can result in normal calcitonin levels in 25–35 % of patients after repeat surgery.

In patients with evidence of recurrent disease, cross-sectional imaging should include the neck (ultrasound), chest (CT), and liver (MRI). Bone scintigraphy and axial skeleton MRI may provide additional information. Remember that radiological evidence of recurrence is unlikely when calcitonin levels are below 250 pg/mL and more likely detected with calcitonin levels more than 500–800 pg/mL. ^{18}F-DOPA PET/CT and ^{18}F-FDG PET/CT have high sensitivity for detection of metastases in patients with calcitonin levels of more than 150 pg/mL (Kauhanen et al. 2011; Beheshti et al. 2009; Ozkan et al. 2011).

Nonsurgical Treatment

Only indicated for palliation/symptom relief:

- *External Beam Radiotherapy*

  Discuss in patients with progressive non-resectable neck disease
  Beneficial for painful bone metastases

- *Systemic Therapies*

  Tyrosine kinase inhibitor – vandetanib
  MIBG/radiolabeled somatostatin analogs
  Within clinical trials:
  Chemotherapy
  Radio immunotherapy with radiolabeled anti-CEA antibodies
  Internal radiotherapy

- *Local Treatments* (lung, liver metastases)

  Radiofrequency ablation
  Chemoembolization

- *Others*

  For symptom control (pain, diarrhea, etc.)
  Somatostatin analogs of some benefit

External beam radiotherapy is of some benefit in patients with advanced MTC in terms of locoregional control but does not appear to improve survival (Martinez et al. 2010).

The use of tyrosine kinase inhibitors in patients with advanced MTC is the subject of much current study. An ongoing randomized phase 3 study of vandetanib with a median follow-up of 24 months has shown significant benefits for treated patients in terms of objective response rates, disease control, and biochemical response; survival analysis is awaited (Wells et al. 2012).

Pearls and Pitfalls

- In patients with elevated postoperative calcitonin who have received less than standard surgical treatment have a low threshold for reoperation.
- The absence of a family history in a patient with MTC does not preclude genetically determined disease.
- Do not operate on a patient with MTC without biochemical proof that there is no pheochromocytoma. The fact that a prior operation was uneventful does not mean the second one will be.
- Up to 25 % of patients with MEN 2A will present with pheochromocytoma as the first manifestation of the syndrome.
- If a patient with MTC is *RET* mutation positive, first-degree relatives should be offered genetic screening.
- Increased serum calcitonin levels can be found in patients without MTC. A pentagastrin stimulation test will be negative in these patients.

References

Beheshti M, Pocher S, Vali R, Waldenberger P, Broinger G, Nader M, et al. The value of 18F-DOPA PET-CT in patients with medullary thyroid carcinoma: comparison with 18F-FDG PET-CT. Eur Radiol. 2009;19(6):1425–34.

Kauhanen S, Schalin-Jantti C, Seppanen M, Kajander S, Virtanen S, Schildt J, et al. Complementary roles of 18F-DOPA PET/CT and 18F-FDG PET/CT in medullary thyroid cancer. J Nucl Med. 2011;52(12):1855–63.

Martinez SR, Beal SH, Chen A, Chen SL, Schneider PD. Adjuvant external beam radiation for medullary thyroid carcinoma. J Surg Oncol. 2010;102(2):175–8.

Ozkan E, Soydal C, Kucuk ON, Ibis E, Erbay G. Impact of (1)(8)F-FDG PET/CT for detecting recurrence of medullary thyroid carcinoma. Nucl Med Commun. 2011;32(12):1162–8.

Wells Jr SA, Robinson BG, Gagel RF, Dralle H, Fagin JA, Santoro M, et al. Vandetanib in patients with locally advanced or metastatic medullary thyroid cancer: a randomized, double-blind phase III trial. J Clin Oncol. 2012;30(2):134–41.

Further Reading

Kloos RT, Eng C, Evans DB, Francis GL, Gagel RF, Gharib H, et al. Medullary thyroid cancer: management guidelines of the American thyroid association. Thyroid. 2009;19(6):565–612.

Chapter 17
Anaplastic Thyroid Cancer

Caroline Connolly and John Glaholm

Definition

Anaplastic, or undifferentiated, thyroid cancer is one of the most aggressive solid tumors with an extremely poor prognosis. It is believed that around 50 % of anaplastic thyroid cancers arise from a prior or coexistent differentiated thyroid carcinoma. The loss of the tumor suppressor gene p53 is an important step in this process.

Incidence

Anaplastic thyroid carcinoma is rare and its incidence is declining (currently 2 per million per year in the USA). It accounts for only 1.6 % of thyroid cancers but is responsible for up to half of all thyroid cancer deaths. It typically presents in the sixth or seventh decade of life and is more common in females.

Presentation

Rapidly enlarging neck mass (80 %)
Dysphagia (40 %)
Hoarse voice (40 %)
Stridor (25 %)
Lymph node mass (50 %)
Systemic symptoms: anorexia, weight loss
Symptoms of metastatic disease: SOB, bony pain, headaches

C. Connolly, MBChB, FRCR (✉) • J. Glaholm
Department of Oncology, Queen Elizabeth Hospital Cancer Centre, Edgbaston,
Birmingham, West Midlands B15 2TH, UK
e-mail: caroline.connolly@uhb.nhs.uk, cconnolly@doctors.org.uk

J.C. Watkinson, D.M. Scott-Coombes (eds.), *Tips and Tricks in Endocrine Surgery*, 143
DOI 10.1007/978-1-4471-2146-6_17, © Springer-Verlag London 2014

Investigations

- Blood tests: Routine biochemistry, bone profile, full blood count, thyroid function, and thyroid autoantibodies.
- Histology: US-guided FNA (accurate in 90 %) or core biopsy. Surgical biopsy may rarely be needed when there is diagnostic uncertainty. It is essential to differentiate anaplastic thyroid carcinoma from thyroid lymphoma or poorly differentiated medullary thyroid cancer as these have a much better prognosis.
- Imaging
  - Staging CT scan of head, neck, chest, and abdomen will give information on local and distant staging. Most commonly metastasizes to the lung.
  - Bone scan: Bone metastases are usually lytic.
  - MRI scan may rarely be needed to assess local infiltration of the neck, particularly if surgery is planned.
  - Radioiodine scanning is not helpful.

Staging (International Union Against Cancer TNM Staging)

- All anaplastic thyroid cancers are considered to be stage IV regardless of size and lymph node status. It should be considered as a systemic disease even if apparently localized.
- T4a: Intrathyroidal and surgically resectable.
- T4b: Extrathyroidal and not surgically resectable.
- IVA: T4a, any N M0.
- IVB: T4b, any N M0.
- IVC: Any T, any N M1.

Histology

Macroscopically: Large unencapsulated invasive cancer with areas of necrosis and hemorrhage.

Microscopically: 3 variants – squamoid, spindle cell, and giant cell.

High mitotic activity is present with necrosis and infiltration.

Areas of well-differentiated thyroid carcinoma are often found concurrently.

Immunohistochemistry: Is an aid to exclude alternative diagnoses. Leukocyte common antigen (lymphoma) and calcitonin (medullary) should be negative.

Molecular pathology: NM23 deletion, p53 mutation common.

Prognosis

Despite multimodality therapy anaplastic thyroid cancer is almost universally fatal. Treatments are aimed at achieving local control and alleviating symptoms. In over 50 % of patients, death results from progressive local disease and upper airway obstruction. Median survival ranges from 7 months for those with localized disease to 3 months in metastatic disease.

Management

The key management approach to this cancer is whether active treatment is appropriate or if palliation is best achieved through symptom control alone. Given its poor prognosis, treatments with high levels of toxicity that are likely to adversely affect quality of life should be avoided, especially in patients with advanced disease. For those patients with localized disease and a good performance status, a combination multimodality approach is likely to give the best chance of local control.

Surgery

As local disease is often very advanced at presentation, the role of radical surgery is limited. Completeness of surgical resection has been identified as a prognostic factor.

If the disease is deemed resectable, then an attempt at total thyroidectomy should be made, with selective resection of regional structures and lymph nodes. Surgery may also be considered after radiotherapy if there is residual local disease.

Surgery plays an important role in palliation, particularly in the prevention of airway compromise and death from asphyxiation. Airway obstruction can occur through 3 mechanisms – external compression of the trachea, intraluminal tumor extension, and bilateral vocal cord paralysis. Tracheostomy plus or minus palliative debulking surgery may be used in those with signs and symptoms of airway compromise.

External Beam Radiotherapy

High-dose radiotherapy may be appropriate in those with inoperable but localized disease with a good performance status. Although a radical dose is aimed for, the treatment is essentially palliative and a compromise may need to be made between adequate dose coverage and toxicity.

Patients should be CT planned and immobilized in a thermoplastic shell. Clinical target volume is the gross tumor volume and involved lymph nodes with a 1 cm margin. Uninvolved locoregional lymph node levels (III, IV, VI, the SCF, and superior mediastinum) should be covered if possible.

Dose – 66Gy in 33 fractions treated over 6.5 weeks.

Intensity-modulated radiotherapy gives the best dose distribution and avoids the critical structures in the neck. An alternative is a two-phase approach, with a first phase consisting of anterior-posterior parallel opposed beams to a dose within cord tolerance, followed by a planned second phase volume including all macroscopic disease.

There may be significant shrinkage during a long course of radiotherapy so replanning during treatment may be necessary. Common toxicities during treatment are skin reaction, mucositis, and esophagitis.

Hyperfractionation with concurrent doxorubicin chemotherapy has shown superior local control rates of around 60 % which improved to over 80 % when combined with surgery.

Adjuvant: EBRT can be used following surgery to prevent or delay local recurrence.

Clinical target volume should cover the entire surgical bed and locoregional lymph node levels III, IV, VI, the SCF, and superior mediastinum.

A postoperative dose of 60Gy in 30 fractions should be achieved if feasible.

Palliative: Most commonly EBRT is used as a palliative measure for temporary relief from local symptoms.

Clinical target volume is all macroscopic disease with a 1 cm margin although this may be compromised to minimize toxicity. Anterior-posterior parallel opposed beams will usually cover this volume adequately.

Dose – 20Gy in 5 fractions.

EBRT is also of use for the palliation of distant disease such as bone and brain metastases.

Radioiodine

Anaplastic thyroid cancers do not concentrate radioiodine; therefore, this has no role in their management.

Chemotherapy

Palliative chemotherapy has poor response rates and is of limited benefit. Single-agent doxorubicin has been used with partial response rates of around 20 %, and combination regimens have failed to show any additional benefit. Paclitaxel has been tested in a phase 2 trial, showing some benefit with response rates of 53 % and a median survival of 32 weeks.

Adjuvant chemotherapy following surgery, commonly with doxorubicin, has been shown to improve outcomes in some retrospective series. More commonly it is used concurrently with radiotherapy to improve local control rates.

Future Treatments

As outcomes remain poor with current standard therapy, patients should be offered clinical trials where available.

Fosbretabulin, a vascular disrupting agent, has shown promise in initial phase 2 clinical trials. Other vascular disrupting agents such as CA4P are also subject to clinical trials.

Pearls and Pitfalls
Pearls

- Palliative approach
- Clinical trials

Pitfalls

- Correct diagnosis
- Failure of local control

Further Reading

Ain KB, Egorin MJ, DeSimone PA. Treatment of anaplastic thyroid carcinoma with paclitaxel: phase 2 trial using ninety-six-hour infusion. Collaborative Anaplastic Thyroid Cancer Health Intervention Trials (CATCHIT) Group. Thyroid. 2000;10(7):587–94.

Bhatia A, Rao A, Ang KK, et al. Anaplastic thyroid cancer: clinical outcomes with conformal radiotherapy. Head Neck. 2010;32(7):829–36.

Haigh PI, Ituarte PH, Wu HS, et al. Completely resected anaplastic thyroid carcinoma combined with adjuvant chemotherapy and irradiation is associated with prolonged survival. Cancer. 2001;91(12):2335–42.

Lim SM, Shin SJ, Chung WY, et al. Treatment outcome of patients with anaplastic thyroid cancer: a single center experience. Yonsei Med J. 2012;53(2):352–7.

Mooney CJ, Nagaiah G, Fu P, et al. A phase II trial of fosbretabulin in advanced anaplastic thyroid carcinoma and correlation of baseline serum-soluble intracellular adhesion molecule-1 with outcome. Thyroid. 2009;19(3):233–40.

Nagaiah G, Hossain A, Mooney CJ, et al. Thyroid cancer: a review of epidemiology pathogenesis, and treatment. J Oncol. 2011;2011:542358.

Patel KN, Shaha AR. Poorly differentiated and anaplastic thyroid cancer. Cancer Control. 2006;13(2):119–28.

Tennvall J, Lundell G, Wahlberg P, et al. Anaplastic thyroid carcinoma: three protocols combining doxorubicin, hyperfractionated radiotherapy and surgery. Br J Cancer. 2002;86:1848–53.

ZYBRESTAT(TM) (CA4P) improves overall survival in a phase 2/3 trial (FACT Study) of patients with Anaplastic Thyroid Cancer (ATC). OXiGENE press release of Phase 2/3 results Sept 2010 posted at http://www.globenewswire.com/newsroom/news.html?d=201261.

Chapter 18
Thyroidectomy Technique

Neil Sharma and John C. Watkinson

Preoperative Considerations

- Always check the patient's recent thyroid function tests (especially important for the toxic patient).
- Ensure preoperative laryngoscopy has been performed and RLN status documented.
- Check consent includes RLN palsy, hypocalcaemia, and hemorrhage.

Marking and Positioning

- Skin is marked for a low anterior neck skin crease incision.
- Marking is best done in the anesthetic room with the patient awake and sitting up (Fig. 18.1).
- Incision is usually 2 cm above the sternal notch.
- When asleep, position the patient supine with a gel roll under the shoulders extending the neck.
- Prep the entire neck to the mandible and laterally to the anterior border of trapezius. Inferiorly clean to the sternal notch.

N. Sharma, MBChB, MRCS, DOHNS (✉)
Department of Otolaryngology, Head and Neck Surgery,
University Hospital North Staffordshire, Newcastle-under-Lyme, UK
e-mail: neil.sharma@outlook.com

J.C. Watkinson
ENT Department, Queen Elizabeth Hospital, Birmingham, UK

J.C. Watkinson, D.M. Scott-Coombes (eds.), *Tips and Tricks in Endocrine Surgery*,
DOI 10.1007/978-1-4471-2146-6_18, © Springer-Verlag London 2014

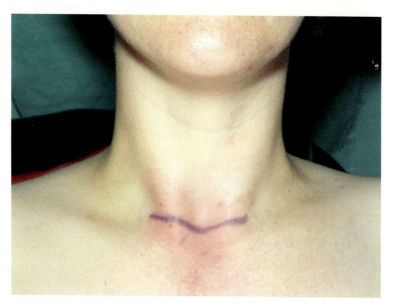

Fig. 18.1 Marking of the neck

Thyroidectomy Technique

Approach to Thyroid Gland

1. Infiltrate the incision area with 1:200,000 adrenaline + Marcaine to give some hydrodissection, hemostasis, and postoperative anesthesia.
2. Raise superior and inferior skin flaps in a sub-platysmal plane to the level of the hyoid superiorly and the suprasternal notch inferiorly.
3. Secure flaps either with sutures or a self-retaining retractor (Joll's).
4. The strap muscles may be separated in the midline (which is a bloodless plane) or divided and retracted. If divided, this is best done deep to sternohyoid, dividing just sternothyroid, allowing access to the upper pole and minimizing the risk of damage to the EBSLN.
5. Dissection may involve sharp dissection, bi-/monopolar diathermy, harmonic scalpel, or a combination of these according to personal/local preferences and training.

Dissection of the Thyroid Gland

1. Enter the paracarotid tunnel and divide the middle thyroid vein.
2. It is often best to start dissection at the superior pole, individually ligating and dividing the vessels.

3. Mobilize the superior pole, exploring Joll's triangle (formed by the midline, strap muscles, and superior pedicle) and identifying and preserving the EBSLN.

   - Care should be taken with the posterior branches of the superior thyroid artery as ligation of these may compromise blood supply to the superior parathyroid gland.

4. For the inferior pole, elevate the muscle and fascia and then individually ligate and divide the inferior thyroid vessels before mobilizing the gland from the anterior surface of the trachea.

5. Dissect the gland medially, taking care to identify the recurrent laryngeal nerve (making up one side of Beahr's triangle, the inferior thyroid artery, and the common carotid artery being the other sides) and both parathyroid glands.

   - Extracapsular dissection may help preserve these structures, allowing the parathyroid glands to be peeled away with their blood supply and the RLN to remain away from the plane of dissection within the fascia.

6. Bleeding vessels in the thyroid bed should be diathermized individually and cautiously to prevent inadvertent damage to the RLN.

7. The ligament of Berry may be dissected with a scalpel to mobilize the thyroid to the junction of the isthmus and the contralateral lobe.

8. If a lobectomy is performed, a clamp is placed across the isthmus and the lobe excised. If a total thyroidectomy is required, a similar dissection is carried out for the contralateral lobe.

Closure

1. Before closing, the parathyroid glands should be inspected to ensure viability (see Chap. 22).

2. Ensure hemostasis using a Valsalva maneuver; be aware of the "triangle of concern," consisting of the RLN, the trachea, and the root of the neck (Fig. 18.2), where small blood vessels have been ligated medial to the nerve. Apply Surgicel® to the thyroid bed.

3. The strap muscles may be approximated by absorbable sutures (if separated in the midline) or re-sutured into position if divided.

4. Consider siting a suction drain in high-risk patients (Graves' disease, extended dissection, bleeding diatheses).

5. Remove the shoulder roll and bring the neck into a neutral position.

6. The platysma may be closed using interrupted absorbable sutures, closing the subcutaneous tissue in the same line.

7. Skin closure is performed according to personal preference, using clips or subcuticular sutures (nonabsorbable/absorbable).

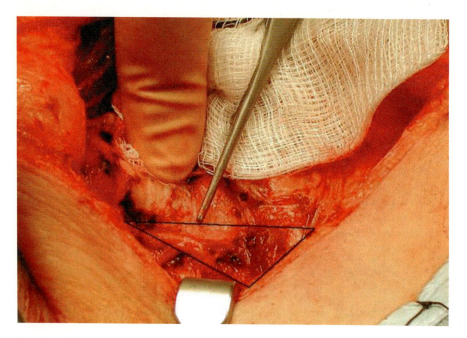

Fig. 18.2 *Triangle* of concern

Postoperative Care

- Following extubation, if there is any concern regarding the airway, then laryngoscopy should be performed prior to the patient leaving the recovery room.
- If clips were used to close the skin, ensure a clip remover is located near to the patient's bedspace to allow rapid removal should the patient develop a hematoma with respiratory embarrassment.
- If a drain was placed, this can generally be removed once output is less than 30 ml over a 24-h period.
- If any voice change is noted, fiber-optic laryngoscopy should be performed prior to discharge and any RLN palsy documented. This should be followed up with a repeat laryngoscopy in the clinic at the first follow-up visit.

Pearls and Pitfalls
Pearls

- Start dissection at the superior pole to facilitate inferior retraction for easier access (essential for retrosternal goiter).
- An accidentally removed parathyroid gland may be reimplanted into the sternocleidomastoid muscle after mincing.

- Medial retraction of the thyroid by the assistant ("creeping") facilitates visualization of the RLN and dissection towards the ligament of Berry.

Pitfalls

- Missing a nonrecurrent inferior laryngeal nerve (0.5–0.8 % incidence on the right side). This and the middle thyroid vein are the only structures in the paracarotid tunnel.
- Failing to ensure hemostasis in the "triangle of concern."
- Injudicious use of diathermy near the RLN.

Recommended Reading

Ecker T, Carvalho AL, Choe JH, Walosek G, Preuss KJ. Hemostasis in thyroid surgery: harmonic scalpel versus other techniques–a meta-analysis. Otolaryngol Head Neck Surg. 2010;143(1):17–25.

Hobbs CGL, Watkinson JC. Thyroidectomy. Surgery. 2007;2010(25):474–8.

Chapter 19
Surgery for Thyrotoxicosis

Sonia Kumar and R. James England

Definition

Hyperthyroidism is characterized by elevated levels of serum thyroxine (T4) and/or elevated levels of serum triiodothyronine (T3) with low levels of thyroid-stimulating hormone (TSH, also known as thyrotropin).

Subclinical hyperthyroidism is characterized by suppressed levels of TSH (<0.5 mU/L) but with levels of T4 and T3 within the normal range.

Thyrotoxicosis is the clinical, physiological, and biochemical state that results from inappropriately high thyroid hormone action on tissues.

Etiology and Incidence

The prevalence of hyperthyroidism is approximately 2 % of the female population with an annual incidence of 2 per 1,000. The most common cause is Graves' disease (GD); other common causes include toxic multinodular goiter (TMNG) and toxic adenoma (TA).

Hyperthyroidism is more common in:

- Women
- Areas of low iodine intake
- Smokers

S. Kumar, MRCS (Eng), DOHNS (✉)
Department of Otolaryngology, Royal Berkshire Hospital, Reading,
London Road Reading, Berkshire RG1 5AM, UK
e-mail: soniakumar111@googlemail.com

R.J. England, MBChB, FRCS (ORL-HNS)
Department of ENT/Head and Neck Surgery, Hull and East Yorkshire NHS Trust,
Castle Hill Hospital, Castle Street, Cottingham, East Riding of Yorkshire HU16 5JQ, UK

J.C. Watkinson, D.M. Scott-Coombes (eds.), *Tips and Tricks in Endocrine Surgery*,
DOI 10.1007/978-1-4471-2146-6_19, © Springer-Verlag London 2014

Causes

- Graves' disease
- Toxic multinodular goiter
- Solitary toxic adenoma
- Rarer causes

  - Thyroiditis

    - Postpartum thyroiditis
    - Acute infection
    - Subacute thyroiditis
    - Traumatic thyroiditis
    - Drug-induced thyroiditis (iodine, amiodarone, lithium, interferon)

  - Thyroid carcinoma
  - Pituitary adenomas
  - Rare: ovarian teratoma, choriocarcinoma, struma ovarii, hydatidiform mole
  - Thyroxine ingestion

Presentation

(see Table 19.1)

Table 19.1 Symptoms and signs of hyperthyroidism

System	Symptoms/signs
Neurological	Restless, nervous, emotional, irritable
	Insomnia
	Tremor
Gastrointestinal	Diarrhea
	Weight loss and increased appetite
Reproductive	Oligomenorrhea/amenorrhea
	Decreased libido
Thyroid	Goiter
Cardiac	Palpitations
	Dyspnea
	Chest pain
	Tachycardia/atrial fibrillation
Dermatological	Thin hair
	Pretibial myoedema/thyroid acropachy
	Palmar erythema
Ophthalmological	Proptosis and exophthalmos
	Lid lag on downward gaze (von Graefe sign)
	Orbital edema and chemosis
	Superficial punctate keratitis, superior limbic keratoconjunctivitis
	Decreased visual acuity, visual field loss, ophthalmoplegia
	Optic nerve compression

Investigations

Assessment of Thyrotoxicosis

- Full history and examination to assess disease severity and comorbidities including age, smoking and family history, dietary history and drug history, HR, BP, weight, and assessment of the neck and ophthalmopathy.
- Assessment of the neck should include examination of the goiter. A palpably dominant nodule should indicate the need for imaging to exclude a solitary toxic adenoma. A bruit on auscultation is pathognomonic of Graves' disease.
- Biochemical evaluation:

  - Serum TSH and free T3 and T4
  - Antibodies: thyroid peroxidase (TPO) (to diagnose hashitoxicosis), thyroid receptor antibodies (TRAbs)(rarely done but elevated in Graves' disease)

- Imaging modalities used in the investigation of thyrotoxicosis depend on the likely treatment plan. In many instances imaging is unnecessary.

  - USS neck: used to differentiate toxic MNG from Graves' disease and thyroiditis
  - Technetium scintigraphy: a rapid noninvasive investigation of particular use in diagnosing a solitary adenoma when neck palpation reveals a dominant nodule

Indications for Surgery

(see Table 19.2)

Preoperative Work-Up

Patients should be rendered euthyroid preoperatively. In cases where this is not possible, patients should be treated with beta-blockers, potassium iodide, or in emergency surgery with corticosteroids.

Table 19.2 Indications for thyroidectomy in the management of thyrotoxicosis

Indications	Contraindications
Symptomatic compression	High surgical risk/comorbidities
Large goiters	1st and 3rd trimesters of pregnancy
Rapid correction of thyrotoxicosis	Uncontrolled thyrotoxicosis (relative
Low uptake of radioactive iodine	contraindication)
Suspected thyroid malignancy	
Coexisting hyperparathyroidism	
Women planning a pregnancy in near future	
Moderate to severe active Graves' ophthalmology	
Pediatric thyrotoxicosis	
Patient choice	

Remember if potassium iodide is used, this reduces thyroid vascularity for a fortnight. After this time a reactive hyperemia occurs (the Jod-Basedow effect)

Intraoperative Considerations

- Most toxic thyroidectomies proceed similarly to nontoxic thyroidectomies and with adequate preparation are not to be feared.
- Total thyroidectomy is the operation of choice unless the toxicosis is caused by a solitary toxic adenoma, in which case total thyroid lobectomy is performed. Subtotal thyroidectomy is no longer the procedure of choice due to the significant proportion of recurrent thyrotoxic patients and the large number of hypothyroid patients with no reduction in surgical side effects.
- Visible pulsation of the anterior jugular veins will normally suggest a thyroid that will "behave toxic."
- Initial mobilization of the gland can be achieved atraumatically by developing a plane between the two strap layers and mobilizing the gland with the deep layer overlying. This also enables assessment of mobility and firmness of the gland without causing bleeding.
- The toxic gland can be friable; surface bleeding is better controlled with bipolar than monopolar diathermy.
- Minimizing intraoperative bleeding will increase the likelihood of parathyroid identification as color contrast will be maintained.
- If bleeding becomes a problem, concentrate on removing the blood supply by dividing the upper pole vessels and the inferior thyroid arterial supply. The latter should be controlled on the gland to optimize the blood supply to the parathyroid glands. If bleeding is still a problem consider isthmusectomy to remove contralateral supply.
- Although the superior parathyroids are normally identified and preserved, do not search for the inferior glands. Instead, ensure they are not adherent to the inferior pole of the thyroid lobe at removal. Searching for them will increase the likelihood of devascularization.
- Remember permanent hypoparathyroidism is generally the result of parathyroid devascularization, not parathyroid removal. Devascularize the thyroid on the gland not distant to it to preserve parathyroid vasculature.

Postoperative Considerations

Thyroid hematoma rates are higher in Graves' disease than in other thyroid pathologies.

Patients undergoing total thyroidectomy should be commenced on the appropriate dose of thyroxine, i.e., *weight (kg) − age (yrs) + 125mcg* (ref).

Serum calcium should be checked postoperatively as per departmental protocol.

Table 19.3 Complications of thyroid surgery

Immediate	Early	Late
Intraoperative bleeding	Hematoma	Hypertrophic/keloid scar formation
Damage to recurrent laryngeal nerve	Seroma	Permanent hypoparathyroidism/
Damage to superior laryngeal nerve	Thyroid storm	hypocalcemia
Thyroid storm	Transient/permanent	
Complications of GA	hypocalcemia	

Complications

(see Table 19.3)

> **Pearls and Pitfalls**
> **Pearls**
>
> - Commonest cause of hyperthyroidism is Graves' disease
> - Total thyroidectomy is the operation of choice (lobectomy for a single functioning adenoma)
> - Minimize intraoperative bleeding
>
> **Pitfalls**
>
> - Inadequate preoperative biochemical control of thyrotoxic state
> - Using monopolar diathermy to control surface bleeding
> - Searching for the inferior parathyroid glands
> - Failure to work with an experienced thyroid anesthetist and to house the patient on a ward used to identifying and treating neck hematoma early

Further Reading

Bahn R, Burch H, Cooper D, Garber J, Greenlee C, Klein I, Laurberg P, et al. Hyperthyroidism and other causes of thyrotoxicosis: management guidelines of the American thyroid association and American association of clinical endocrinologists. Thyroid. 2011;21(6):593–646.

Bartalena L, Baldeschi L, Dickinson AJ, Eckstein A, Kendall-Taylor P, Marcocci C, Mourits MP, Perros P, Boboridis K, Boschi A, Currò N, Daumerie C, Kahaly GJ, Krassas G, Lane CM, Lazarus JH, Marinò M, Nardi M, Neoh C, Orgiazzi J, Pearce S, Pinchera A, Pitz S, Salvi M, Sivelli P, Stahl M, von Arx G, Wiersinga WM. Consensus statement of the European group on Graves' orbitopathy (EUGOGO) on management of Graves' orbitopathy. Thyroid. 2008;18:333–46.

Hannan A. The magnificent seven: a history of modern thyroid surgery. Int J Surg. 2006;4:187–91.

Kang AS, Grant CS, Thompson GB, van Heerden JA. Current treatment of nodular goiter with hyperthyroidism (Plummer's disease): surgery versus radioiodine. Surgery. 2002;132:916–23.

Palit TK, Miller 3rd CC, Miltenburg DM. The efficacy of thyroidectomy for Graves' disease: a meta-analysis. J Surg Res. 2000;90:161–5.

Chapter 20
Retrosternal Goiter

Neil Sharma and John C. Watkinson

Definition

- Enlargement of the thyroid beyond the thoracic inlet occurs in between 5 and 20 % of goiters. The terminology varies between retrosternal, substernal, intrathoracic, and mediastinal.
- Retrosternal goiter was originally described as being a goiter in which greater than 50 % of the thyroid was below the thoracic inlet.
- Currently, there is controversy as to what the definition should be and consequently there is variability in the literature.
- The most frequently used definitions are:

  Any part of the thyroid below the thoracic inlet
  A thyroid reaching the aortic arch
  A thyroid reaching the level of T4
  50 % of the thyroid below the thoracic inlet

Incidence

- The incidence of retrosternal goiter is between 0.2 and 45 % of all cases of thyroid enlargement depending on the definition used.
- It is usually a multinodular goiter with both cervical and mediastinal extension; true primary mediastinal goiter is rare.

N. Sharma, MBChB, MRCS, DOHNS (✉)
Department of Otolaryngology,
Head and Neck Surgery, University Hospital North Staffordshire,
Newcastle-under-Lyme, UK
e-mail: neil.sharma@outlook.com

J.C. Watkinson
ENT Department, Queen Elizabeth Hospital, Birmingham, UK

J.C. Watkinson, D.M. Scott-Coombes (eds.), *Tips and Tricks in Endocrine Surgery*,
DOI 10.1007/978-1-4471-2146-6_20, © Springer-Verlag London 2014

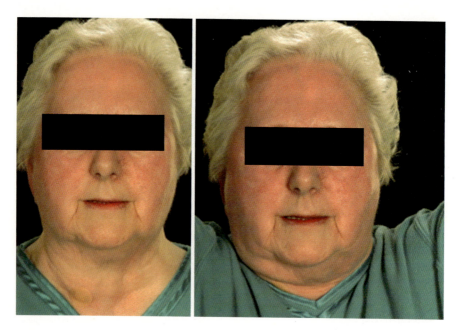

Fig. 20.1 Pemberton's sign. The presence of a retrosternal goiter causes facial flushing and distended superficial veins. Mild flushing is noted with the arms by the side indicating some baseline obstruction at rest

Presentation

Retrosternal goiters may present as for any other thyroid enlargement, and the presence of retrosternal extension may sometimes only be elicited by observing other symptoms and signs.

Indicators of Compression

- Stridor
- Dysphagia
- Tracheal narrowing
- Esophageal compression
- SVC syndrome

Other Indicators of Retrosternal Goiter

- Pemberton's sign (facial flushing, distended neck and head superficial veins, inspiratory stridor, and elevation of JVP when the arms are raised above the head) (Fig. 20.1)

Fig. 20.2 Coronal MRI scan of a patient with retrosternal goiter. This patient had palpable, laterally displaced neck vessels suggesting benign disease (Berry's sign), thyroid cork sign (tracheal deviation to the side of the cervical thyroid swelling (*left*) indicating a hidden (*right*) retrosternal goiter), and incidental dextrocardia

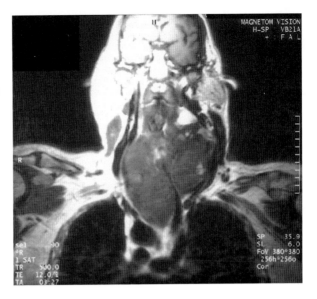

- Thyroid cork (deviation of the trachea to the same side as a cervical goiter, due to contralateral retrosternal thyroid enlargement)
- Berry's sign (inability to feel the carotid pulse when the vessels are displaced laterally by the goiter suggests malignancy) (Fig. 20.2)

Investigations

As for thyroid disease confined to the neck, patients should have:

- Blood tests: TSH, free T4 and T3, thyroid antibodies, and calcium
- FNAC if possible (this may be facilitated by ultrasound)

Prior to surgery more detailed imaging and functional studies may be needed to determine the extent of retrosternal extension and the relation of the thyroid to the structures in the mediastinum:

- Magnetic resonance imaging
- Computed tomography (with or without contrast)
- Respiratory flow loop testing (in patients with compressive symptoms, this may help to predict postoperative tracheomalacia)

The goiter may be recurrent and it is important to check that the patient does not have a vocal cord palsy.

Medical Management

- Should the patient be hyperthyroid, liaison with an endocrinologist is essential, and indeed, this may have been the referral source.
- Treatment with thionamides may help to render the patient euthyroid and beta-blockers may aid with symptom control.
- Radioiodine treatment can be useful to reduce the size of the goiter which may serve to improve compressive symptoms and make any future surgery less difficult in the infirm.

Indications for Surgery

Absolute Indications

- Clinical or radiological evidence of significant or life-threatening compression
- Proven malignancy

Relative Indications (These Relate to the Asymptomatic Retrosternal Goiter)

- Less clear-cut.
- Have generated significant debate over the past few years (see further reading).
- The risk of malignancy in a goiter not amenable to FNA and the risk of airway compromise are cited in favor of uniform thyroidectomy.
- The lack of evidence and the often elderly age of patients with low likelihood of malignancy are used as arguments to justify a conservative approach.

Tips for Surgery

Preoperative

- Preoperative planning including adequate anatomical mapping of the goiter (via chest radiograph and CT/MRI) is essential.
- In all cases where difficulty is expected, the opinion of a thoracic surgeon should be sought and their expertise available during the operation if needed.

Operative

- Many retrosternal goiters can be safely removed via a cervical incision, but the presence of distorted anatomy or an ectopic intrathoracic thyroid may necessitate a sternotomy. In these cases, the thyroid may still be delivered via a cervical approach by experienced thyroid surgeons; otherwise, a thoracic approach may be necessary.
- Whichever incision is chosen, it is important that appropriate access is obtained. Make an adequate incision and remember, *the lower the goiter, the higher the cut*. Access can be improved by dividing the strap muscles, especially for very low, bilateral goiters.
- When approaching the gland, begin with the easier side and ligate the upper pole first. Stay within the pseudocapsule and work medial to lateral. Ensure you are in the correct plane for the lower pole vessels and always get control inferiorly.
- Some advocate the use of vessel sealing devices to reduce the risk of bleeding and ease the removal of the gland.

Postoperative

- The patient should be nursed on a ward accustomed to managing post-thyroidectomy patients and, if a sternotomy was necessary, have access to nursing staff used to managing these wounds.
- Some patients may benefit from a monitored bed on a high dependency/intensive care unit for at least the first postoperative night.

Complications and Outcomes

Recent studies report no increase in complication rates for patients with retrosternal goiter. This may be due in part to more stringent selection for surgery as well as the acceptance that the majority of these goiters will be successfully delivered via the neck. A summary of complications is given in Table 20.1.

Table 20.1 Complications of surgery for retrosternal goiter

Early complications	Intermediate complications	Late complications
Hemorrhage	Infection	Permanent hypocalcemia
Tracheomalacia	Hypocalcemia	Poor scar
Pleural injury	Poor healing	Permanent RLN palsy
Mediastinal injury		Complications of sternotomy
RLN palsy		
Hypocalcemia		

Due to the lack of large studies and usually indolent nature of the disease, the available evidence on recurrence rates is limited. Previously, it was usual practice to perform subtotal thyroidectomy which confers greater risk of recurrence than for total procedures. For patients in whom intrathoracic thyroid issue was left, it is important to ensure they are regularly followed up, using cross-sectional imaging where necessary to monitor the size of the residual thyroid tissue.

Pearls and Pitfalls
Pearls

- Most retrosternal goiters are benign
- The majority can be dealt with via a cervical approach
- Ensure an adequate incision
- Have a good assistant

Pitfalls

- Poor preoperative imaging
- Making an inadequate incision
- Lack of appropriate postoperative monitoring (airway compromise and other compressive symptoms)

Further Reading

Hardy RG, Bliss RD, et al. Management of retrosternal goitres. Ann R Coll Surg Engl. 2009;91(1):8–11.

Randolph GW, Shin JJ, et al. The surgical management of goiter: part II. Surgical treatment and results. Laryngoscope. 2011;121(1):68–76.

Rugiu MG, Piemonte M. Surgical approach to retrosternal goitre: do we still need sternotomy? Acta Otorhinolaryngol Ital. 2009;29(6):331–8.

Shaha AR. Substernal goiter: what is in a definition? Surgery. 2010;147(2):239–40.

Chapter 21
Lymph Node Surgery for Thyroid Cancer

Neil Sharma and Ashok Shaha

Background

- The thyroid has a dense network of intraglandular lymphatics which joins collecting and draining lymphatic trunks and leaves the gland with the vascular supply. This results in early multifocal disease and significant locoregional spread.
- Nodal disease is usually ipsilateral but may be bilateral (30 %).

Table 21.1 Lymph node levels of the neck

Level	Nodes
Lateral compartment	
I	Submental and submandibular nodes
II	Deep cervical nodes from the skull base to the level of the hyoid. Further divided by the relationship to the accessory nerve (level 2a being medial and 2b lateral)
III	Deep cervical nodes from the level of the hyoid to the cricoid
IV	Deep cervical nodes from the level of the cricoid to the suprasternal notch
V	Posterior triangle nodes can be divided by their relationship to a plane drawn through the level of the cricoid cartilage (Va is above and Vb is below the accessory nerve)
Central compartment	
VI	Pre- and paratracheal nodes from the level of the hyoid bone above to the sternal notch below and the carotid artery laterally
Mediastinal compartment	
VII	Superior mediastinal nodes as far as the superior aspect of the brachiocephalic vein

N. Sharma, MBChB, MRCS, DOHNS (✉)
Department of Otolaryngology, Head and Neck Surgery,
University Hospital North Staffordshire,
Newcastle-under-Lyme, UK
e-mail: neil.sharma@outlook.com

A. Shaha
Jatin P. Shah Chair in Head and Neck Surgery and Oncology,
Memorial Sloan-Kettering Cancer Center,
New York, USA

J.C. Watkinson, D.M. Scott-Coombes (eds.), *Tips and Tricks in Endocrine Surgery*,
DOI 10.1007/978-1-4471-2146-6_21, © Springer-Verlag London 2014

Table 21.2 Lymph node staging

NX	Regional lymph nodes cannot be assessed
N0	No regional lymph node metastasis
N1	Regional lymph node metastasis
N1a	Metastasis in level VI (pretracheal and paratracheal, including prelaryngeal and Delphian lymph nodes)
N1b	Metastasis in other unilateral, bilateral, or contralateral cervical or upper/superior mediastinal lymph nodes

Used with the permission of the American Joint Committee on Cancer (AJCC), Chicago, Illinois. The original source for this material is the *AJCC Cancer Staging Manual*, Seventh Edition (2010) published by Springer Science and Business Media LLC, www.springer.com

- Lymph node metastases to the regional lymph nodes are relatively common in PTC and occur early on; the incidence of palpable neck disease is between 15 and 40 % (40–90 % have occult disease).
- Metastases from follicular carcinoma are less common (<20 %).
- Recurrent disease in lymph nodes accounts for 60–75 % of all neck recurrences.
- Elderly patients and those with bilateral and mediastinal disease have a poorer prognosis.

Lymphatic Drainage of the Thyroid

Lymph node groups at the highest risk of metastases from DTC are in the central compartment (level VI), the lower jugular chain (levels III and VI), and the lower posterior triangle (level Vb) (Fig. 21.1).

Major drainage:

- Middle jugular nodes – level III
- Lower jugular nodes – level IV
- Posterior triangle nodes – level Vb

Minor drainage:

- Pretracheal and paratracheal nodes – level VI
- Superior mediastinal nodes – level VII

Assessment of Lymph Nodes

Clinical Examination

- Detailed clinical examination is essential.
- Important factors to document are:

Fig. 21.1 Lymph node levels of the neck (Reproduced with permission from Watkinson JC, Gilbert RW, Arnold H, editors. Stell and Maran's textbook of head and neck surgery and oncology. 5th ed. London: Hodder Arnold; 2012. p. 433, Fig 23.12)

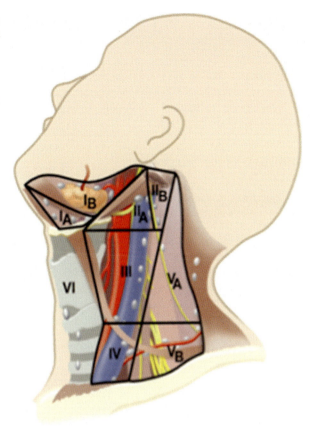

- Number, approximate size, and location of lymph nodes
- Consistency of nodes (firm, soft, cystic, etc.)
- Skin changes (including tethering)

Imaging

- *Ultrasound*: Factors suggesting malignancy include increased size, cystic change, calcification, hyperechogenicity, peripheral/mixed vascularity, and a more rounded shape.
- *CT/MRI*: Enlarged, multiple nodes may be evident, and note should be taken of central necrosis, cystic change, dense cortical enhancement more than that of muscle, and calcification, all of which may indicate metastases. The superior mediastinum may also be assessed and this allows for accurate pre-operative staging.

Cytology

- *FNAC*: May be diagnostic for metastatic thyroid cancer. The presence of thyroglobulin in the sample is strongly predictive of metastatic thyroid tissue.
- *Biopsy*: Occasionally diagnosis may be made following the open removal of a lymph node for another reason (e.g., suspicion of lymphoma).

Indications for Surgery

Central Neck Dissection

Prophylactic: Level VI dissection should be performed in high-risk patients (male, >45 years of age, tumor size >4 cm, extracapsular/extrathyroidal disease) and in those in whom lateral neck disease is present.

Therapeutic: If nodes are apparent preoperatively or encountered intraoperatively, central neck clearance should be performed.

On-table ultrasound may be used to assess level VI/VII lymph nodes intraoperatively.

Level VI may be further subdivided into VIA (medial to the RLN) and VIB (lateral to the RLN).

- For small cancers in low-risk patients, a level VIA dissection should be performed, with significantly lower risk to the RLN than a full-level VI clearance.

Lateral Neck Dissection

- There is no role for prophylactic lateral neck dissection.
- Preoperatively confirmed lateral neck lymph node disease warrants a selective neck dissection (levels IIa–Vb), with preservation of the accessory nerve, sternocleidomastoid muscle, and internal jugular vein.
- Suspicious nodes in the lateral neck found during surgery may be assessed by FNAC or frozen section, with selective neck dissection being indicated should the biopsy confirm metastasis. A central compartment clearance should also be carried out in these cases.
- The presence of ipsilateral lymph node disease necessitates the examination of the contralateral neck, with suspicious nodes being examined using FNAC or frozen section and neck dissection being undertaken should they be positive.
- Advanced disease may require a more extensive neck dissection, involving levels I and/or Va, if necessary sacrificing surrounding structures (sternocleidomastoid muscle, internal jugular vein, or skin).

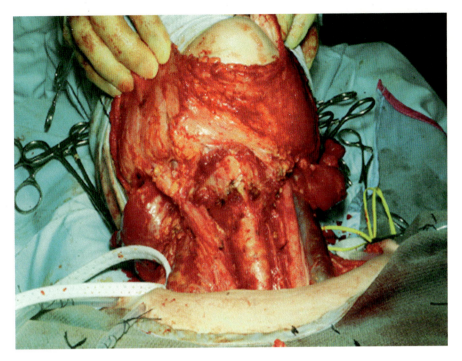

Fig. 21.2 Anterior view of the neck following central and lateral neck dissection

Surgical Considerations

Lymph node metastases are often multiple; therefore, surgery should consist of selective neck dissection of at-risk levels rather than "berry picking."

Central Neck Dissection

- This is usually performed with a total thyroidectomy as an extension of extracapsular dissection.
- Full central compartment clearance involves all node-bearing tissue from the hyoid bone to the sternal notch and laterally to the carotid sheath (Fig. 21.2).
- Involved lymph nodes are more frequent in the inferior compartment; therefore, superior dissection may be less aggressive, thus aiding preservation of the superior parathyroid glands on their blood supply.

Procedure

- Skeletonize the RLN from its superior aspect at the cricothyroid joint to the sternal notch and carefully elevate it from the surrounding tissues, avoiding traction.

- Dissect lymph nodes from the IJV laterally to the trachea medially (passing under the RLN)
- Inferiorly, dissect any thymic tissue along with adjacent lymph nodes/fatty tissue in level VI.
- It may be necessary to reimplant the inferior parathyroid glands if their blood supply has been compromised during dissection.

Lateral Neck Dissection

- The lateral neck may be accessed via an extended Kocher's incision or an extended superior thyroid incision at the level of the cricoid cartilage.
- Levels I, IIb, and Va are less frequently involved; therefore, a selective lateral neck dissection incorporating levels IIa to Vb is usually sufficient, unless there is extensive disease in which case a modified radical neck dissection should be employed.
- Suarez's fat pad can be located between levels IIa and IIb.

Procedure

- Working laterally to medially, identify levels II to V.
- Identify the accessory nerve.
- The lower end of the sternocleidomastoid muscle may be divided and retracted caudally to facilitate access to level IV.
- Dissect levels IIa, III, IV, and Vb, preserving the internal jugular vein, phrenic nerve, and brachial plexus.
- In high-risk cases, level IIb can be dissected along with Suarez's fat pad.
- Should there be extension into surrounding structures, they should be excised in continuity.

Complications

- Central neck dissection is associated with an increased risk of RLN damage and both temporary and permanent hypoparathyroidism.
- The brachial plexus, phrenic, vagus, and hypoglossal nerves are at risk but should not be damaged in routine cases.
- Chyle leak may complicate lateral neck dissection and should be repaired.
- Neuropraxia of the accessory nerve may occur due to ischemia resulting from traction but usually recovers.
- Some branches of the cervical plexus may be divided with relatively little morbidity.

Controversies

- An alternative to formal neck dissection is to identify the sentinel lymph node using methylene blue and sending the node for frozen section, with the presence or absence of malignancy determining whether to proceed with clearance. However, this violates level VI and is therefore not recommended.

Pearls and Pitfalls

Pearls

- If nodal disease is suspected preoperatively, ensure adequate imaging to include the neck up to the skull base and inferiorly to the superior mediastinum
- Divide the sternocleidomastoid to ensure full access to level IV, the carotid sheath, and Chassaignac's triangle
- Levels I and Va are not usually involved in LN metastases and do not need to be routinely dissected

Pitfalls

- "Berry picking" suspicious nodes instead of performing formal neck dissection
- Failing to adequately clear level Vb

Recommended Reading

British Thyroid Association and Royal College of Physicians. Guidelines for the management of thyroid cancer. In: Perros P, editor. Report of the Thyroid Cancer Guidelines Update Group. London: Royal College of Physicians; 2007.

Carty SE, Cooper DS, et al. Consensus statement on the terminology and classification of central neck dissection for thyroid cancer. Thyroid. 2009;19(11):1153–8.

Cooper DS, Doherty GM, et al. Revised American Thyroid Association management guidelines for patients with thyroid nodules and differentiated thyroid cancer. Thyroid. 2009;19(11):1167–214.

Stack BC Jr, Ferris RL, et al. American Thyroid Association Surgical Affairs Committee. American Thyroid Association consensus review and statement regarding the anatomy, terminology, and rationale for lateral neck dissection in differentiated thyroid cancer. Thyroid. 2012;22(5):501–8.

Chapter 22
Complications in Thyroid Surgery and How to Avoid Them

M.A. Alzahrani and Gregory W. Randolph

Complications in Thyroid Surgery and How to Avoid Them

- Although the current incidence of complications of thyroid surgery in good hands is acceptably low, the impact of complications can be significant.
- Literature clearly shows a direct correlation between experience and rate of complications, a finding that supports a dedicated subspecialty training.

Hematoma

- Incidence is low (0–3 %).
- Typically results from venous bleeding from small veins.
- Usually presents during the initial 4–8 h postoperative period but may have a delayed presentation up to several days, which makes it challenging to make an evidence-based recommendation regarding length of "safe" hospital stay.
- Current literature shows no significant value of placing drains after thyroid surgery, and pressure dressing does not seem to prevent hematoma formation.
- Venous pressure can be reduced during and after surgery by obtaining reverse Trendelenburg position (head and back up).
- At the conclusion of the procedure and prior to closure, a final check for hemostasis should be confirmed by asking the anesthetist to perform a Valsalva maneuver which increases the venous pressure. This should be performed with a careful reinspection of the operative field.

M.A. Alzahrani • G.W. Randolph, MD (✉)
Otolaryngology – Head and Neck Surgery,
Massachusetts Eye and Ear Infirmary,
243 Charles St., Boston, MA 02114, USA
e-mail: gregory_randolph@meei.harvard.edu

J.C. Watkinson, D.M. Scott-Coombes (eds.), *Tips and Tricks in Endocrine Surgery*,
DOI 10.1007/978-1-4471-2146-6_22, © Springer-Verlag London 2014

- Acceptable means of controlling vessels include appropriate application of ligatures, clips, bipolar diathermy, and other energy technologies such as the harmonic scalpel.
- Additional use of hemostatic agents (e.g., Surgicel) at the thyroid bed may be helpful but should never be a substitute for strict hemostasis.
- When encountered, a hematoma should urgently be addressed by early securing of the airway (ideally by intubation), securing of hemostasis, and evacuation of the hematoma.
- A small nonprogressive hematoma can be expectantly managed.
- A large and progressive hematoma carries a major risk of airway obstruction that results from blood accumulating in a closed space leading to ecchymotic submucosal laryngeal edema. This process could result in a progressive airway narrowing which makes intubation potentially difficult if not performed on a timely fashion. Prompt attention to the airway, preferably by means of endotracheal intubation, with concurrent evacuation of hematoma and achievement of hemostasis should be performed.
- Postoperative care should be optimized to avoid nausea, vomiting, and coughing.
- Instructions should be given to nurses in order to alert the physician about any concerns of neck swelling or breathing or swallowing difficulties.

Recurrent Laryngeal Nerve (RLN) Injury

- Incidence of RLN injury varies and may be small in expert hands. However, rates of immediate RLN paralysis after surgery are likely in the order of 5–10 % in the general community.

Preoperative Considerations

- A detailed knowledge of RLN anatomy is essential.
- Pre- and postoperative voice does not correlate well with the actual status of RLN. Therefore, pre- and postoperative direct laryngeal exam should routinely be employed on all thyroid patients.

Intraoperative Considerations

- Thyroid surgery should ideally be done by an expert with the aid of magnification loupes and with the adjunct of intraoperative neural monitoring (IONM).

- There are three main objectives that constitute the rationale behind endorsing routine IONM in thyroid surgery:

  1. Identification of the nerve: by "neural mapping" of the trajectory of RLN.
  2. Aid in dissection: dissection at difficult areas by intermittently stimulating tissues that are being dissected.
  3. Prognostication of postoperative function: visual assessment remains insufficient in identifying nerve injury. Some studies demonstrated that only 10 % of nerve injuries can be appreciated by visual inspection.

- The surgeon should also be capable of performing the different surgical approaches to the RLN when appropriate. There are generally three approaches for the RLN:

  1. The lateral approach: it is ideal during routine thyroidectomy, in which the RLN is identified at the level of midpole of the thyroid after the superior or inferior poles are dissected. Robust medial retraction of the thyroid lobe is the key that widely exposes the lateral thyroid region. One can use the inferior edge of the thyroid cartilage's inferior cornu and the point of crossing of RLN and the inferior thyroid artery as landmarks.
  2. Inferior approach: This approach identifies the RLN at the thoracic inlet, at the apex of the RLN triangle. It is ideal to carry out during revision surgery.
  3. Superior approach: This approach is ideal in cases of large and substernal goiters as the RLN's most superior segment remains almost always constant just proximal to the laryngeal entry point.

- Systematic stepwise approach during thyroidectomy positively impacts the outcome.
- Maintaining a bloodless field is critical to recognition of parathyroid and RLN.
- Blind clamping and/or cautery significantly places RLN at risk of injury and should always be avoided.
- Tissue bands that are transparent can safely be divided.
- Prior to clamping or dividing a less transparent tissue band, dragging the neural monitor along the ventral and dorsal aspects practically nullifies the risk of inadvertent nerve injury.
- At the inferior pole, the RLN typically runs deep to the inferior thyroid artery (ITA). However, do not assume a constant relationship between the RLN and the inferior thyroid artery as it can be very variable and may vary from side to side.
- Use of monopolar diathermy or harmonic scalpel adjacent to the RLN should be avoided, whereas transient precise use of fine-tipped bipolar diathermy is well tolerated.
- When the goiter is lobulated and has clefts or the tubercle of Zuckerkandl is disproportionately enlarged, the RLN can assume a position between clefts or a ventrally displaced position which places it at a significantly higher risk of injury. Neural monitoring may prove very helpful in these cases.
- During medial retraction of the lobe, the RLN should be maintained under view as significant tension could result in neuropraxic damage to the nerve.
- RLN typically runs deep to the ligament of Berry. It, however, may assume a position between the leaflets of the ligament and this has to be ruled out prior to clamping or dividing.

- If oozing is encountered, which frequently happens at the RLN-Berry's ligament interaction, better visualization is first restored by gentle gauze pressure or pledgets soaked in diluted epinephrine solution.
- A nonrecurrent RLN can be at a higher risk of injury, and neural monitoring is helpful in early identification by demonstrating a signal with shorter latency of the vagus nerve at the level of thyroid cartilage and a negative signal lower down after the RLN branches off the vagus.

External Branch of the Superior Laryngeal Nerve (SLN)

- Can be visually identified in 80 % and electrically in 100 % of cases.
- It runs inferomedially along the lateral surface of the sternothyroid muscle.
- Stimulation of the external branch of the SLN results in an electromyographic (EMG) activity and a visible contraction of the cricothyroid muscle at the anterolateral larynx.
- A robust landmark for SLN is the oblique line of the thyroid cartilage where the inferior constrictor inserts.
- Dragging the neural monitor along the superior pole bands to be divided can prove very helpful in avoiding SLN injury.
- Visualization can be facilitated by downward mobilization of the superior thyroid pole using a clamp.
- Ligation of the superior thyroid vessels close to the capsule is generally safe in avoiding injury to SLN
- Care should be practiced as the SLN may assume a lower position that interacts with superior thyroid vessels.
- In cases of significant enlargement of the superior pole, visualization can be achieved by transecting the laryngeal head of the sternothyroid muscle as it hoods the superior pole. Doing this is inconsequential.

Hypoparathyroidism

- It can be transient (lasting <6 months) or permanent.
- Transient hypoparathyroidism occurs in up to 20 % of patients undergoing total thyroidectomy, and it results from the surgical manipulation as the parathyroids are peeled off the thyroid capsule.
- Permanent hypoparathyroidism is still being reported with an incidence of 1–2 %, and it results from devascularization of or inadvertent removal of parathyroids.

Preoperative Considerations

- Knowledge of parathyroid embryology and anatomy is essential in recognizing these tiny organs that can be situated from the mandible down to the mediastinum.

Intraoperative Considerations

- Dissecting the thyroid at the immediate extracapsular plane is a key principle to preserve parathyroids and their blood supply.
- Parathyroids are visually identified by their brown-reddish tan color, discrete edge, and the gliding motion when the surrounding fat is manipulated.
- Inferior parathyroid is typically found within 1 cm from the inferior thyroid pole and can be reflected inferolaterally with its intact pedicle.
- Extensive dissection to identify the entire course of RLN can interfere with parathyroid blood supply that extends from lateral to medial and is better avoided. Instead, RLN can be visualized in a skip fashion.
- Superior parathyroids are typically found with 1 cm from the cricothyroid articulation and less commonly at a descended location near the RLN-inferior thyroid artery interaction.
- If the parathyroid appears after dissection nonviable or dusky, autotransplantation (after mincing it in small pieces) in the ipsilateral sternocleidomastoid muscle is undertaken.
- A final careful inspection of the thyroid specimen is highly encouraged looking for parathyroid glands. If found, it can be autotransplanted at the ipsilateral sternocleidomastoid muscle.

Postoperative Considerations

- All patients undergoing bilateral thyroid surgery should ideally be monitored for hypocalcemia in recovery room and every 8 h for the first postoperative day, although many units have individual protocols for post-thyroidectomy patients.
- Initial mild hypocalcemia (Ca ≥8.5 mg/dl, 2.10 mmol/l) can be safely managed by watchful observation.
- Hypocalcemia with minimal symptoms (perioral numbness) can be treated with oral calcium supplement and vitamin D.
- More significant symptoms usually require intravenous calcium.

Further Reading

Evans SR. Surgical Pitfalls, prevention and management. Philadelphia: Saunders; 2009.

Gopalakrishna Iyer N, Shaha AR. Complications of thyroid surgery: prevention and management. Minerva Chir. 2010;65(1):71–82.

Kennedy SA, et al. Meta-analysis: prophylactic drainage and bleeding complications in thyroid surgery. J Otolaryngol Head Neck Surg. 2008;37(6):768–73.

Randolph GW. Surgery of the Thyroid and Parathyroid Glands. Philadelphia: Saunders; 2012.

Randolph GW, et al. Electrophysiologic recurrent laryngeal nerve monitoring during thyroid and parathyroid surgery: international standards guideline statement. Laryngoscope. 2011;121 Suppl 1:S1–16.

Chapter 23
Revision Thyroid Surgery

Ram Moorthy and Neil Tolley

Definition

- Revision thyroid surgery is defined as second surgery on the thyroid or the central thyroid bed.

Indications

- It encompasses a wide range of procedures for benign or malignant thyroid pathology (Table 23.1). It can be same side or contralateral to previous surgery.

Incidence

- Incidence is between 5 and 19 % (Alesina et al. 2008; Scott-Coombes et al. 2009).

R. Moorthy, FRCS (ORL-HNS) (✉)
Otolaryngology- Head and Neck Surgery, ENT,
Heatherwood and Wexham Park Hospitals NHS Trust,
Wexham Park Hospital, Wexham Street,
Wexham Berkshire SL2 4HL, UK
e-mail: ram.moorthy@rammoorthy.co.uk, rammoorthy@mac.com

N. Tolley, MD, FRCS
Department of Otolaryngology, Head and Neck Surgery,
Imperial College Healthcare NHS Trust, St Mary's Hospital,
Praed St, London W2 1NY, UK

J.C. Watkinson, D.M. Scott-Coombes (eds.), *Tips and Tricks in Endocrine Surgery*,
DOI 10.1007/978-1-4471-2146-6_23, © Springer-Verlag London 2014

Table 23.1 Reasons for revision surgery

Recurrent thyrotoxicosis
Recurrent compressive symptoms for a MNG
Completion surgery for cancer
Locoregional cancer recurrence
Review or change in pathological diagnosis
New pathology (hyperparathyroidism)

Table 23.2 Pathological and surgical factors influencing revision surgery

Avoidable pathological factors	Avoidable surgical factors
Error in cytological diagnosis	Inappropriate primary procedure
Error in pathological diagnosis	Inadequate primary procedure, a correct preoperative diagnosis should direct the correct primary surgical strategy
Unavoidable pathological factors	Unavoidable surgical factors
Completion of thyroid surgery based on pathology	New or recurrent pathology
Failure to make a preoperative diagnosis	

Minimizing Rate of Revision Thyroid Surgery

- Revision surgery can be reduced by correctly managing pathological and surgical factors at the time of their primary surgery (Table 23.2).

Complications

- Complications of revision surgery are higher particularly in inexperienced, low-volume surgeons.
- Recurrent laryngeal nerve injury is more likely if revision surgery is undertaken on the same side as previous surgery (14 %) compared to the contralateral side (3.2 %) (Table 23.3) (Scott-Coombes et al. 2009).

Preoperative Work-Up

- Surgery should preferably be undertaken by high-volume surgeons.
- Review pathological and cytological diagnosis in a thyroid MDT meeting.
- Preferably review previous operation record. Specifically seek information about the procedure performed, identification of the RLN, and parathyroid glands.
- Preoperative vocal cord assessment is mandatory.

Table 23.3 Complications of revision surgery (Alesina et al. 2008; Scott-Coombes et al. 2009; Bergenfelz et al. 2008; Cappellani et al. 2008; Kronz and Westra 2005; Kupferman et al. 2002; Lefevre et al. 2007; Menegaux et al. 1999; Mishra and Mishra 2002; Randolph et al. 2011; Robert 2005; Watkinson 2010; Wu et al. 2011)

	Primary surgery	Revision surgery
Recurrent laryngeal nerve injury		
Temporary	1.8–4.8 %	1–4.1 %
Permanent	0.4–4.0 %	1.2–5.4 %
Hypocalcemia		
Temporary	9.9–32.3 %	5–14.8 %
Permanent	1.0–17.3 %	2.5–15.5 %
Bleeding	0.9–2.1 %	0.7–3.5 %
Infection	1.6 %	0.2 %

- Repeat cross-sectional imaging may be indicated to facilitate surgical planning.
- The aim in the majority of patients is to undertake a total or completion thyroidectomy.

Operative Technique

- Nerve monitoring can aid both identification and dissection of the RLN in scar tissue.
- The previous incision should be used.
- The procedure may be executed by a conventional midline or lateral approach.
- Expose the strap muscles in the midline and laterally to the sternomastoid muscle.

Conventional midline approach	Lateral approach
Strap muscles are separated in midline. The trachea is a useful guide because the midline raphe may have already been disrupted during original surgery	After dissection of the plane between the strap muscles and sternomastoid muscle, the great vessels are identified and the thyroid gutter opened down to the prevertebral plane
The contralateral lobe or thyroid gland remnant is identified and exposed by careful dissection of the strap muscles	The inferior and superior attachments of the sternothyroid muscle are divided to provide access to the thyroid, and the assistant retracts the tissues medially
The superior thyroid pedicle, if present, is identified and ligated close to the gland to minimize risk of damage to the ELN	The parathyroid glands, RLN and ELN are identified and thyroid vessels are ligated
Ligation of middle thyroid vein if present	Dissection continues from lateral to medial dividing Berry's ligament thereby mobilizing the thyroid remnant or lobe
Identify recurrent laryngeal nerve and parathyroid glands. Dissect the thyroid remnant free of the nerve, ligating the inferior thyroid pedicle, if required	The thyroid is removed from its final medial attachment to the trachea

Postoperative Instructions

- Carefully observe the neck for swelling and airway compromise.
- Monitor postoperative calcium.
- Patient is discharged once serum calcium is in the normal range.
- Depending upon the surgeons preference, remove skin sutures between 2 and 5 days.

Summary

- Revision surgery cannot be avoided, but it can be reduced.
- Surgical approach is determined by previous surgery, the proposed procedure, and surgical experience.

Pearls and Pitfalls
Pearls

- Revision surgery cannot be avoided, but it can be reduced
- Surgical approach is determined by previous surgery, the proposed procedure, and surgical experience
- Surgery should be undertaken by high-volume surgeons
- Pre- and postoperative laryngoscopy are mandatory
- Try to avoid a subtotal technique
- Cancer in the vast majority of patients should be a preoperative diagnosis

Pitfalls

- Failing to follow the correct surgical strategy
- Failing to fully review previous pathology
- Adopting a subtotal technique

References

Alesina P, Rolfs T, Walz M. Reoperative surgery for benign thyroid diseases. Pol J Surg. 2008; 80:441–5.

Bergenfelz A, Jansson S, Kristoffersson A, et al. Complications to thyroid surgery: results as reported in a database from a multicenter audit comprising 3,660 patients. Langenbecks Arch Surg. 2008;393:667–73.

Cappellani A et al. The recurrent goiter: prevention and management. Roma: Luigi Pozzi; 2008.

Lefevre JH, Tresallet C, Leenhardt L, Jublanc C, Chigot J-P, Menegaux F. Reoperative surgery for thyroid disease. Langenbecks Arch Surg. 2007;392:685–91.

Kronz JD, Westra WH. The role of second opinion pathology in the management of lesions of the head and neck. Curr Opin Otolaryngol Head Neck Surg. 2005;13:81–4.

Kupferman ME, Mandel SJ, DiDonato L, Wolf P, Weber RS. Safety of completion thyroidectomy following unilateral lobectomy for well-differentiated thyroid cancer. Laryngoscope. 2002;112:1209–12.

Menegaux F, Turpin G, Dahman M, et al. Secondary thyroidectomy in patients with prior thyroid surgery for benign disease: a study of 203 cases. Surgery. 1999;126:479–83.

Mishra A, Mishra SK. Total thyroidectomy for differentiated thyroid cancer: primary compared with completion thyroidectomy. Eur J Surg. 2002;168:283–7.

Randolph GW, Shin JJ, Grillo HC, et al. The surgical management of goiter: part II. Surgical treatment and results. Laryngoscope. 2011;121:68–76.

Robert LW. Recurrent laryngeal nerve electrophysiologic monitoring in thyroid surgery: the standard of care? J Voice. 2005;19:497–500.

Scott-Coombes D, Kinsman R, Walton P. The British Association of Endocrine and Thyroid Surgeons. Third National Audit Report London: BAETS; 2009.

Watkinson JC. Fifteen years' experience in thyroid surgery. Ann R Coll Surg Engl. 2010;92:541–7.

Wu G, Pai SI, Agrawal N, Richmon J, Dackiw A, Tufano RP. Profile of patients with completion thyroidectomy and assessment of their suitability for outpatient surgery. Otolaryngol Head Neck Surg. 2011;145:727–31.

Further Reading

Agarwal G, Aggarwal V. Is total thyroidectomy the surgical procedure of choice for benign multinodular goiter? An evidence-based review. World J Surg. 2008;32:1313–24.

Ashok RS. Revision thyroid surgery, technical considerations. Otolaryngol Clin North Am. 2008;41:1169–83.

Frable WJ. Surgical pathology–second reviews, institutional reviews, audits, and correlations: what's out there? Error or diagnostic variation? Arch Pathol Lab Med. 2006;130:620–5.

Franc B, de la Salmoniere P, Lange F, et al. Interobserver and intraobserver reproducibility in the histopathology of follicular thyroid carcinoma. Hum Pathol. 2003;34:1092–100.

Johnson S, Goldenberg D. Intraoperative monitoring of the recurrent laryngeal nerve during revision thyroid surgery. Otolaryngol Clin North Am. 2008;41:1147–54.

Kim MK, Mandel SH, Baloch Z, et al. Morbidity following central compartment reoperation for recurrent or persistent thyroid cancer. Arch Otolaryngol Head Neck Surg. 2004;130:1214–6.

Mitchell J, Milas M, Barbosa G, Sutton J, Berber E, Siperstein A. Avoidable reoperations for thyroid and parathyroid surgery: effect of hospital volume. Surgery. 2008;144:899–907.

Pai SI, Tufano RP. Reoperation for recurrent/persistent well-differentiated thyroid cancer. Otolaryngol Clin North Am. 2010;43:353–63.

Richer SL, Wenig BL. Changes in surgical anatomy following thyroidectomy. Otolaryngol Clin North Am. 2008;41:1069–78.

Shemen L, Oh A, Turner J. Reoperative thyroid surgery. Oper Tech Otolaryngol. 2003;14:106–8.

Sosa JA, Bowman HM, Tielsch JM, Powe NR, Gordon TA, Udelsman R. The importance of surgeon experience for clinical and economic outcomes from thyroidectomy. Ann Surg. 1998;228:320–30.

Stalberg P, Svensson A, Hessman O, Akerstrom G, Hellman P. Surgical treatment of Graves' disease: evidence-based approach. World J Surg. 2008;32:1269.

Chapter 24
Extended Surgery for Extra-thyroidal Disease Invasion

Ajith Paulose George and Maninder Singh Kalkat

Definition

- Extra-thyroid extension (ETE) relates to invasion of thyroid tumor beyond its capsule into local and regional structures, T3–T4a and T4b (7th E^{dn} TNM) classification.
- Tumor may extend directly from the thyroid itself or from extracapsular spread of involved lymph nodes.
- ETE occurs in anaplastic, medullary, and differentiated thyroid cancer (DTC) and is the most important prognosticator of outcome from a surgical perspective in the latter.
- The risk factors for ETE (age >45, size of tumor >4 cm, and metastatic disease) are similar to those associated with poor prognosis in DTC.

Incidence

- The reported incidence of DTC with ETE ranges from 5 to 34 %.
- Reported 5-year survival rates with thyroid cancer invading the upper aerodigestive tract are 70–80 %.

A.P. George, MBChB, FRCS (ORL-HNS) (✉)
Department of Otolaryngology, Head and Neck Surgery,
Russells Hall Hospital, Dudley, West Midlands, Birmingham Heartlands Hospital, UK
e-mail: georgea288@aol.com, ajithgeorge@nhs.net

M.S. Kalkat, FRCS
Department of Thoracic Surgery, Birmingham Heartlands Hospital, UK
e-mail: mkalkat@gmail.com

J.C. Watkinson, D.M. Scott-Coombes (eds.), *Tips and Tricks in Endocrine Surgery*,
DOI 10.1007/978-1-4471-2146-6_24, © Springer-Verlag London 2014

Table 24.1 Signs and symptoms of ETE

	Structure	"T" stage	Symptom/signs
Central neck	Strap muscles	T3	Hard fixed thyroid mass
	Parathyroids	T3	–
	Skin	T4a	Skin ulceration/erythema
	RLN and SLN	T4a	Dysphonia or weak fatigable voice, stridor
	Trachea and Larynx	T4a	Hemoptysis, stridor, cough
	Esophagus	T4a	Dysphagia
	Prevertebral fascia	T4b	Neck stiffness
Lateral neck	IJV	T4b	Radiological diagnosis
	Carotid	T4b	Radiological diagnosis
	Sternocleidomastoid	T4b	Lateral neck mass
	Phrenic, X, XI	T4b	Raised hemidiaphragm, dysphonia, stiff shoulder

Presentation

- Most patients present asymptomatically; thus, a high index of suspicion for ETE is required.
- When considering possible presenting signs and symptoms (Table 24.1), it is useful to appreciate central and lateral structures in the neck that may be involved with ETE (Fig. 24.1).

Investigations

- All patients require fiber-optic pharyngolaryngoscopy to examine for intraluminal disease.
- CT and MRI with contrast evaluate potential laryngeal cartilage involvement, intraluminal extension, and tracheal, esophageal, and vascular involvement.
- The use of iodine contrast in CT delays postoperative radioactive iodine (RAI) scanning for residual or metastatic disease.
- Ultrasound is useful for evaluating minimal ETE into strap muscles and has variable reported results for detecting either tracheal or esophageal involvement, 42.9 and 28.6 %, respectively.
- Be aware of non-RAI avid tumors (see section "Medical Management"). In this case if the thyroglobulin is high, FDG PET-CT is more likely to show metastatic disease, as these tumors are metabolically active with high glucose uptake.
- Barium swallow may show a mucosal esophageal lesion.
- Bronchoscopy and esophagoscopy should be undertaken in patients suspected to have ETE to assess mucosal involvement.
- Lung function studies may be appropriate in patients with upper aerodigestive tract involvement who may be candidates for partial laryngectomy.

Fig. 24.1 Patterns of thyroid and extra-thyroid extension (*green* T1, *blue* T2, *purple* T3, *orange* T4a, and *black* T4b) (Reproduced with permission from Rubin P, Hansen JT. TNM staging atlas. Philadelphia: Lippincott Williams & Wilkins; 2007. p. 91, Fig 12.1)

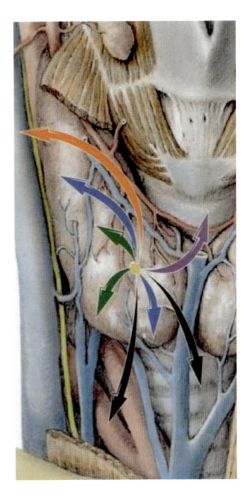

- Preoperative speech and swallowing assessments help with intraoperative decision making in terms of recurrent laryngeal nerve (RLN) resection, partial laryngectomy, and vocal cord augmentation.

Medical Management

- By definition all DTC with ETE is treated by adjuvant RAI (ATA 2009 & BTA 2007).
- There is no primary role for medical management in medullary thyroid cancer. Patients treated with adjuvant external beam radiotherapy (EBRT) have been shown to have poorer survival though this may reflect the severity of the disease being treated.

- Certain histological subtypes of DTC associated with poor RAI avidity respond poorly to this treatment. In these cases, surgical clearance of disease macroscopically is paramount ± adjuvant EBRT:
  - Trabecular
  - Tall cell
  - Insular
  - Poorly differentiated

- New research into chemotherapeutic agents such as deacetylase inhibitors and peroxisome proliferator-activated receptor-γ (gamma) agonists may improve sensitivity to RAI.
- Both the American Thyroid Association and British Thyroid Association (ATA and BTA) have outlined recommendations for ERBT in T4 disease in ages over 45 and over 60, respectively, if there is gross residual disease after surgery. EBRT is not recommended in T3 disease though some studies suggest a possible benefit in the over 60s.

Tips for Surgery

Preoperative

- Knowledge and appreciation of the extent of possible ETE is important for surgical planning.
- Be prepared to open the chest if mediastinal disease is anticipated.
- A key recommendation in the BTA guidelines is that a surgeon should have training and expertise in the management of thyroid cancer and be a member of the MDT.
- Surgery offers the most effective option to reduce an individual's risk of disease recurrence and mortality from ETE related problems. The principles are:
  - To remove gross tumor
  - Preserve function
  - Preserve vital structures
  - Use adjuvant therapies

- It is important to discuss preoperatively with the patient the possibility of sacrificing vital structures for tumor clearance.

Operative

Strap Muscle Invasion

- Strap muscles are the most commonly involved sites for ETE due to their anatomical proximity, but involvement is not associated with poorer outcomes.
- Management consists of wide local excision obtaining negative margins. Consequently there is no reported increased comorbidity due to the loss of the strap muscles.

Recurrent Laryngeal Nerve

- Recurrent laryngeal nerve involvement may be direct tumor involvement or pressure on the nerve by surrounding tumor extension.
- Preoperative function determines the intraoperative management plan:
    - *Nerve paralyzed and involved in tumor* – en bloc resection.
    - *Presence of a functioning nerve* – If sparing the nerve comes at a cost of leaving behind gross volume tumor, then this should be avoided. It is imperative to check the contralateral nerve is disease free prior to resection. In bilateral nerve involvement, steps should be taken to preserve at least one nerve that would result in the least amount of gross tumor volume left behind. An attempt should be made to peel off the nerve from the tumor.
- There is no overall survival benefit in studies where the nerve is sacrificed versus preservation with RAI.
- Intraoperative monitoring of the nerve has been shown to be beneficial in decision making between sacrificing or peeling off the nerve.
- If the nerve is sacrificed, then consider early medialization for patients who are less likely to compensate and are at greater risk of aspiration.
- When the nerve is sacrificed, consider greater auricular nerve reconstruction primary anastomosis and arytenoid adduction, all of which are superior to leaving patients untreated.

Laryngeal Involvement

- Though the laryngeal perichondrium is an ineffective barrier against the invasion of thyroid carcinoma, the larynx is less frequently involved.
- Tumor invasion limited to laryngeal cartilage can be dealt with shaving off the tumor. The airway is not breached and function remains preserved.
- The intraluminal spread of tumor is usually limited to one side of the larynx and is amenable to partial or hemi-laryngectomy.
- Total laryngectomy or more complex procedures may be required in some cases.

Trachea

- Invasion of the trachea accounts for 50 % of deaths and occurs in a third of cases of ETE.
- Anterior or lateral invasion is the most common route of spread.
- Tumor invades the cartilage rings and through intercartilaginous spaces into the tracheal lumen.
- Tumor limited to tracheal cartilage can be shaved off, provided complete clearance can be ensured. This can be evaluated by frozen section.
- In the event of tumor invading full thickness of trachea, it is prudent to resect the involved trachea and perform end-to-end anastomosis. The results of tracheal

resection and reconstruction have improved significantly and carry minimal morbidity in expert hands. About 4 cm of trachea can be resected without requiring release procedures to attain tension-free anastomosis.
- Removing small patch of tracheal wall and wedge resections can compromise oncological resection and is associated with postoperative complications, including dehiscence and stenosis.
- When inoperable, endoscopic tumor ablation with Nd:YAG LASER followed by electrocoagulation is reportedly well tolerated.

Esophagus

- Esophageal involvement is found in one fifth of patients.
- Esophageal mucosa is resistant to direct invasion; thus, disease is usually confined to the muscular coat sparing the mucosa.
- The use of a bougie intraoperatively to define the mucosa allows for disease clearance without entering the esophagus. The tumor is dissected off the mucosa developing submucosal plane with blunt dissection. Tears in the mucosa are repaired primarily and buttressed with muscle flaps.
- A full-thickness involvement of a smaller area can be excised and a tension-free closure performed and covered with muscle flap.
- Circumferential resections require reconstruction with interposition of pedicled, fascial, or fasciocutaneous flaps or gastric, colonic, or jejunal transfer, the latter being the recommended procedure.
- Stents can be used for palliation.

Neck Vessels

- Both the carotid artery and internal jugular veins should be preserved where possible.
- In the interest of macroscopic disease clearance, unilateral resection of the IJV may be necessary as per a comprehensive neck dissection.
- Carotid artery involvement is a contraindication to surgery.

Complication and Outcomes

- Complications of tracheal reanastomosis include hypoparathyroidism, mediastinitis, anastomotic dehiscence, VCP, and death.
- Following central compartment clearance for ETE, there is an increased risk of hypoparathyroidism and seroma.
- The patients' outcome is dependent on the success of surgical resection.
- Implications of extra-thyroidal disease:

- Increased incidence of local and distant metastatic disease
- Increased risk of local recurrence
- Region-specific complications of involved structures
- Decreased overall survival

Pearls and Pitfalls
Pearls

- ETE can present asymptomatically with no clinical signs
- ETE has the greatest negative impact on prognosis
- Leaving macroscopic disease to preserve RLN function has no detrimental impact on survival or disease recurrence
- "Shave procedures" are effective in managing ETE in the absence of intra-luminal involvement

Pitfalls

- The use adjuvant RAI should not excuse poor macroscopic surgical clearance of disease, and its success is determined by histological subtypes
- Surgery for ETE is highly specialized and should preferably be undertaken by those skilled in the procedures mentioned above
- Not all elements of ETE are correlated with poorer survival; thus, management should be performed on a case-by-case basis depending upon the specific structures involved and the degree to which they are affected
- There is a poor correlation between change in voice and the presence of vocal cord paralysis

Chapter 25
Managing the Airway in Thyroid Surgery

Scott Russell

Introduction

Despite expectations, management of the airway in thyroid surgery is rarely a problem.

When problems do occur, however, they can be at any stage of the operation.

Preoperative Assessment

It should be remembered that these patients are at risk of difficult intubation for the same reasons as those presenting for non-thyroid surgery and should be assessed as such. However, the presence of a compressive mass in the neck and mediastinum provides additional problems.

History

- The history may indicate difficulty breathing, especially when lying down, suggestive of significant compression.
- History of a sense of difficulty swallowing is not of diagnostic use regarding the airway. Choking when trying to swallow, however, may well indicate significant compression.

S. Russell
Department of Anaethestics,
Queen Elizabeth Hospital, Birmingham, UK
e-mail: scott.russell@uhb.nhs.uk

J.C. Watkinson, D.M. Scott-Coombes (eds.), *Tips and Tricks in Endocrine Surgery*,
DOI 10.1007/978-1-4471-2146-6_25, © Springer-Verlag London 2014

- Other aspects of the history may indicate recurrent laryngeal nerve damage, particularly a change of voice. A past history of thyroid surgery, or other surgery in the neck, may be of significance, especially if resulting in change of voice. If the thyroid mass is malignant, there is a possibility of invasion of the nerve.

Examination

- The apparent size of the goiter may be misleading as the mass normally extends posteriorly and inferiorly.
- Stridor may be present, although this is rare.
- Tracheal deviation may also be visible, although the utility of this observation is questionable.

Investigations

- CT or MRI scan of the neck is most useful in assessing the site and degree of obstruction.
- AP or PA chest radiograph is less useful as the compression is usually anteroposterior.
- Flow volume loops will predictably usually show some degree of extra-thoracic large airways obstruction.
- Thyroid function tests will indicate thyrotoxicosis. These should ideally be normal before surgery. In some cases this will not be possible, and surgery may need to proceed with less than ideal control. Blood loss and hemodynamic instability should be expected in these circumstances.
- If free thyroxine levels are raised due entirely to overtreatment with thyroxine, this does not lead to problems intraoperatively, as manipulation of the gland does not lead to sudden large increases in plasma level of the hormone.

Intubation

- Special care should be taken in planning airway management, as emergency tracheotomy is likely to be very difficult in these patients.
- Intravenous induction, inhalational induction, and awake fiber-optic intubation are all possible.
- In the vast majority of patients, preoxygenation, intravenous induction, demonstration of ability to manually ventilate the lungs, and subsequent neuromuscular blockade followed by oral tracheal intubation is perfectly safe.

- Extrinsic compression is easily bypassed by the tracheal tube, although a smaller-than-usual tube may be a wise measure. The tip of the tube is usually well beyond the compression. It is wise to ensure that the tube is passed well into the trachea, both for this reason and also because of the risk of it being displaced into or even out of the larynx by airway manipulation during surgery. A reinforced tube is recommended because of the risk of kinking of the tube during these manipulations.
- Where there is significant compression, especially with stridor, neuromuscular blockade should not be administered until the airway has been secured. Inhalational induction, while often the recommended approach in cases of difficult airway, may be difficult in these cases because the turbulent airflow caused by the obstruction may make the process very slow. If the patient is agreeable, awake fiber-optic intubation is the safest and easiest approach.

Extubation

- The immediate concern on extubation is laryngospasm due to recurrent laryngeal nerve damage.
- Meticulous pharyngeal toilet should be applied before extubation to reduce the risk of laryngospasm from other causes.
- Previous practice was to extubate the patient while deeply anesthetized but breathing spontaneously and to observe the cords by direct laryngoscopy to check for bilateral movement. This practice is now less common:

  - Laryngoscopy in the non-paralyzed patient, even carried out with meticulous care, does not necessarily give an ideal view of the cords and can cause morbidity (cut lips, damaged teeth).
  - Unilateral cord palsy is unlikely to lead to immediate surgical intervention, and subsequent observation can be by fiber-optic nasendoscopy as appropriate.
  - If there is concern about bilateral damage, after bilateral surgery or with pre-existing damage to the contralateral cord, then this technique can still be used, although there is a good argument for fiber-optic visualization of the cords in the still-anesthetized patient.

- In the case of unexpected severe laryngospasm, it will be necessary to re-anesthetize the patient and administer a short-acting muscle relaxant (suxamethonium):

  - The patient should be reintubated and other causes of laryngospasm sought.
  - Once breathing spontaneously and sufficiently deeply anesthetized, the patient should be extubated under direct visualization of the larynx.
  - If bilateral severe laryngospasm again occurs, suggesting bilateral cord damage, reintubation should be performed. It will then be necessary to create a formal surgical tracheostomy.
  - Return of cord function over subsequent days can then be checked by fiber-optic laryngoscopy.

- The other postoperative airway concern is of surgical hemorrhage into the neck. This can cause airway obstruction secondary to submucosal vocal cord edema from obstruction of the local veins in the neck. This may be life threatening and will require surgical evacuation of the hematoma. Immediate decompression by opening the wound may be lifesaving. Attempts to assess the airway fiber-optically may precipitate total obstruction and should only be carried out where the facilities for immediate tracheotomy exist. Usually this should be done in the operating theater.

Pearls and Pitfalls
Pearls

- Work with a regular anesthetist to develop local expertise.
- Cross-sectional imaging with 3-D reconstruction can provide a preoperative "road map."
- Regional anesthesia helps to minimize the chances of increased venous pressure at the time of reversal of anesthesia.

Pitfalls

- Ignore stridor at your peril.
- Indirect vocal cord inspection at the time of extubation is not a reliable method of assessing vocal cord function.

Chapter 26
Voice Change Following Thyroid and Parathyroid Surgery

Jeremy Davis and Meredydd Harries

Definition

- Some temporary voice change following thyroid or parathyroid surgery is common (up to 30 %).
- Permanent change occurs in around 10–15 % of thyroid operations.
- There is controversy over the definition of "permanent" – but voice change persisting more than 12 months after surgery is most common definition.
- Mild changes in voice may not require any active management. The need for intervention often depends on the occupation of the patient.
- Where thyroid or parathyroid surgery results in a change in voice, it is usually an adverse change. However, occasionally, the voice may be improved.
- A normal subjective postoperative voice does not exclude the presence of nerve damage.

Causes

- Local mechanical (direct, traction) or thermal nerve damage at operation. Nerves at risk are:-
  - Recurrent laryngeal. Note that around 40% of laryngeal nerves bifurcate before they enter the larynx and in these the motor fibers are probably in the anterior branch. Be aware of anatomical variations including early bifurcation and the importance of identifying the nerve in all cases.

J. Davis, MBBS, FRCS (✉)
ENT Department, Medway Maritime Hospital, Gillingham, Kent ME5 8NY, UK
e-mail: jeremy.davis@nhs.net

M. Harries
Department of Otolaryngology, Head and Neck Surgery,
Royal Sussex County Hospital, Eastern Road, Brighton BN2 5BE, UK
e-mail: meredlolharries@hotmail.com

J.C. Watkinson, D.M. Scott-Coombes (eds.), *Tips and Tricks in Endocrine Surgery*,
DOI 10.1007/978-1-4471-2146-6_26, © Springer-Verlag London 2014

- External branch of the superior laryngeal nerve.
- Pharyngeal nerve plexus.

- Secondary to the thyroid/parathyroid pathology, e.g., tumor infiltrating nerve and pressure on nerve. There are usually preoperative voice changes.
- Effect of intubation on larynx including localized edema and dislocation of the arytenoid cartilage.
- Direct or indirect trauma to local tissues, e.g., stretching/incision of strap muscles and postoperative scarring.
- Hypothyroidism following surgery without adequate hormonal replacement.
- Functional (psychogenic) dysphonia related to the surgery or the underlying diagnosis – this is rare.

Effects

- While many patients may be totally unaware of or tolerate minor temporary voice change, in some there will be significant adverse effects on the quality of life and/or the ability to continue in employment. This is especially true of occupations with considerable voice use (professional voice users) and patients who sing either professionally or as a hobby.
- Bilateral vocal cord palsy is rare but can occur. There is usually immediate stridor in recovery and urgent treatment is required.

Surgeon's Legal Responsibilities

All surgeons undertaking thyroid and/or parathyroid surgery should ensure that:

- Patients are counseled about the risk of temporary or permanent voice change. The majority of thyroid and parathyroid surgery is elective (planned) surgery, and this allows counseling to take place well before the date of surgery.
- This should be documented in the written preoperative consent record.
- Laryngeal examination is undertaken preoperatively and (especially if there is any postoperative voice change) after surgery.

It is good practice for all surgeons to undertake an ongoing audit of their own practice so they are aware of how many of their own patients have voice change postoperatively.

Prevention

- Meticulous surgery aimed at minimizing trauma to nerves.
- Consider laryngeal nerve monitoring in selected cases (e.g., revision surgery). However, there is no current evidence that this reduces the incidence of neural damage and voice change.
- There is greater risk of damage in cases of malignancy and revision surgery.

Assessment

- Stridor occurring immediately after surgery should always be investigated without delay by direct fiberoptic laryngeal examination. If the patient has a preexisting contralateral nerve palsy, then stridor can occur following hemithyroidectomy – this is one reason why preoperative laryngoscopy must always be performed.
- Patient's reports of voice change are reliable. Postoperative care (both immediate and at subsequent outpatient follow-up) should include direct questioning about voice change which can be quantified with the use of specific voice questionnaires.
- Laryngoscopy or videostroboscopy may show abnormalities related to recurrent laryngeal nerve injury (unilateral paralysis or paresis) or those related to superior laryngeal nerve injury (arytenoid asymmetry, epiglottis skewed, asymmetrical mucosal wave, and difference in height of the two vocal cords).
- Superior/external laryngeal nerve damage can also be demonstrated by viewing the larynx as the patient goes from low to high frequency as the posterior glottis rotates towards the side of the paralysis – due to the lack of cricothyroid action on that side.
- EMG assessment of the superior laryngeal nerve, Voice Handicap Index, Voice-Related Quality of Life and Vocal Performance Questionnaires, and the GRBAS (grade or severity (G), roughness of the voice (R), breathiness (B), asthenia (A), and strain (S)) perceptual rating of voice quality are mainly used to document voice before and after surgery in research projects looking at voice change after neck surgery.
- EMG may have a prognostic role in identifying regeneration and the timing and necessity of voice surgery.

Treatment

Immediate

- If a recurrent laryngeal nerve is accidentally transected at operation, it should be repaired at that time using microsurgical techniques. Although full recovery is unlikely, some degree of reinnervation and synkinesis may allow medialization of the paralyzed cord and an acceptable voice.
- Immediate stridor resulting from bilateral vocal fold palsy is a surgical emergency and should be treated without delay. This is usually accomplished by reintubation and subsequent tracheostomy.
- Temporary vocal fold lateralization can sometimes be performed if the surgical team has the correct skill mix, avoiding tracheostomy. A suture is placed around the vocal cord and then tightened externally to allow cord lateralization to establish an acceptable airway.

Later

- Voice change not related to bilateral vocal cord paralysis can usually be managed conservatively at first. Most voice change following thyroid surgery will spontaneously resolve within three months due to:

  - Recovery of temporary nerve damage (neuropraxia) and other surgical trauma to the surrounding tissues.
  - Spontaneous compensation where there is permanent damage but a phonatory gap of less than 1 mm.

- If the voice remains adversely changed at three months after operation, then the patient should be referred to a multidisciplinary voice team.
- If a recurrent laryngeal nerve has been sacrificed (as may sometimes be necessary when treating thyroid cancer) or accidentally transected at surgery (whether or not it is repaired), earlier referral to a multidisciplinary voice team is indicated.
- The multidisciplinary voice team will assess the patient. The type and timing of treatment will depend on many factors including the degree of lateralization of the paralyzed cord and the occupation and vocal handicap of individuals.
- In selected cases phonosurgical intervention may be indicated including vocal cord medialization (using thyroplasty or vocal fold injection) and/or arytenoid adduction techniques.
- Surgery to improve the voice will often help as long as patient selection is good, but is unlikely to restore the voice completely to its preoperative quality.
- The timing of surgery depends on the degree of disability, but ideally it should be more than 4 months after the initial thyroid or parathyroid surgery which caused the problem.
- In permanent bilateral vocal cord paralysis, partial laser resection of the vocal process of the arytenoid can give a sufficient airway and is very successful. This is usually done at a later stage if there is no recovery of movement, but carries a small risk of aspiration and poor voice.
- Laryngeal reinnervation – from local nerves including the ansa cervicalis and split phrenic remains controversial but may offer an alternative to standard phonosurgical techniques.

Pearls and Pitfalls
Pearls

- Voice change is common – your patients need to know this
- Prevention is better than cure – take care when dissecting close to nerves
- Most voice change is temporary
- Identify significant voice changes and refer to voice specialist team

Pitfalls

- Do not miss stridor secondary to bilateral laryngeal palsy
- Do not ignore patients with postoperative voice change
- Be realistic when counseling patients preoperatively
- Perform preoperative laryngoscopy in all patients

Further Reading

Kandil E, Abdelghani S, et al. Motor and sensory branching of the recurrent laryngeal nerve in thyroid surgery. Surgery. 2011;150(6):1222–7.

Marina MB, Marie JP, Birchall MA. Laryngeal reinnervation for bilateral vocal fold paralysis. Curr Opin Otolaryngol Head Neck Surg. 2011;19(6):434–8.

Meek P, Carding PN, et al. Voice change following thyroid and parathyroid surgery. J Voice. 2007;22(6):765–72.

Rubin AD, Sataloff RT. Vocal fold paresis and paralysis: what the thyroid surgeon should know. Surg Oncol Clin N Am. 2008;17(1):175–96.

Soylu L, Ozbas S, et al. The evaluation of the causes of subjective voice disturbances after thyroid surgery. Am J Surg. 2007;194(3):317–22.

Stojadinovic A, Shaha AR. Prospective functional voice assessment in patients undergoing thyroid surgery. Ann Surg. 2002;236(6):823–32.

Chapter 27
Postoperative Management of Thyroid Cancer

Beng K. Yap

Definition

- Differentiated thyroid carcinoma refers to both papillary and follicular thyroid carcinomas arising from thyroid follicular epithelium.

Early Postoperative Period

- Following total or near total thyroidectomy, patient should be started on liothyronine (T3). The usual adult dose is 20 mcg tds.
- Serum calcium should be checked within 24 h of surgery. Start calcium supplementation if patient is hypocalcemic according to local protocols.

Role of Radioiodine Ablation (RAI)

- The use of radioiodine-131 (I^{131}) to destroy residual normal thyroid tissue following total or near total thyroidectomy is known as radioiodine remnant ablation (RAI).
- The radioiodine "therapy" is a term refers to I^{131} administration to treat recurrent or metastatic disease.

B.K. Yap, MBChB, FRCP, FRCR
Department of Clinical Oncology,
The Christie NHS Foundation Trust, Wilmslow Road,
Withington, Manchester, Lancashire M20 4BX, UK
e-mail: beng.yap@christie.nhs.uk

J.C. Watkinson, D.M. Scott-Coombes (eds.), *Tips and Tricks in Endocrine Surgery*,
DOI 10.1007/978-1-4471-2146-6_27, © Springer-Verlag London 2014

Table 27.1 Indication for postoperative RAI based on the American Thyroid Association (ATA) guideline

TNM stage	Description	I[131] Decreased risk of death	I[131] Decreased risk of recurrence	May facilitate initial staging and follow-up	RAI usually recommended
T1a	≤1 cm, intrathyroidal, microscopic multifocal	No	No	Yes	No
T1b	1–2 cm intrathyroidal	No	Conflicting data[a]	Yes	Selective use[a]
T2	>2–4 cm intrathyroidal	No	Conflicting data[a]	Yes	Selective use[a]
T3	>4 cm				
	≤45 years old	No	Conflicting data[a]	Yes	Yes
	>45 years	Yes	Yes	Yes	Yes
	Any size, any age, minimal extrathyroid extension	No	Inadequate data[a]	Yes	Selective use[a]
T4	Any size with gross extrathyroidal extension	Yes	Yes	Yes	Yes
Nx, N0	No metastatic nodes documented	No	No	Yes	No
N1	≤45 years old	No	Conflicting data[a]	Yes	Selective use[a]
	>45 years old	Conflicting data[a]	Conflicting data[a]	Yes	Selective use[a]
M1	Distant metastasis	Yes	Yes	Yes	Yes

[a]Because of either conflicting or inadequate data, ATA cannot recommend either for or against RAI ablation for this entire subgroup. However, selected patients within this subgroup with higher-risk features may benefit from RAI ablation

- The rationale of RAI are:

    1. To eradicate all residual normal thyroid cells including potential microscopic cancer cells
    2. To facilitate early detection of recurrence based on serum thyroglobulin (Tg) measurement and radioiodine scanning during follow-up period
    3. To provide reassurance to patients by the knowledge of undetectable Tg and negative radioiodine scanning which imply that all thyroid tissue has been destroyed

Indications for Postoperative RAI

The indication for postoperative RAI based on the American Thyroid Association (ATA) guideline (Cooper et al. 2009) is summarized in Table 27.1.

Table 27.2 Example of low-iodine diet

Do eat	Try not to eat
Fresh and frozen fruit and vegetables	Seafood and fish
Fresh and frozen meats	Dairy product: cow's/goat's milk, cheese, ice cream, yoghurt, and butter
Rice, pasta, and potatoes	Egg yolks
Soft drinks, fruit juices, beer, wine, tea, coffee, and soya milk	Some cough mixtures and health foods (such as seaweed, kelp, cod liver oil, vitamins, and mineral supplements) contain iodine. If the label lists iodine, do not take the supplement while on this diet
Plain fats and oils (nondairy)	Avoid food from restaurants, fast-food chains, and takeaways
Olive oil spread	
Fresh and home-made bread	
The best way to make sure of the iodine content is to prepare your food from fresh ingredients yourself	
Do not add any of the ingredients listed in the other box	
Table salt with no added iodine may be used	

Preparation for Radioiodine Ablation or Therapy

- Patient should adopt a low-iodine diet (see example in Table 27.2) for 2 weeks prior to RAI ablation or I^{131} or therapy and avoid sources of excess iodine such as:

  1. Iodine-based contrast for CT scanning (defer I^{131} for 2–3 months after iodine contrast)
  2. Amiodarone (defer I^{131} for 4–6 months after amiodarone withdrawal)

- I^{131} uptake is thyroid-stimulating hormone (TSH) dependent.
- I^{131} can be administered within 3–4 weeks of thyroidectomy if RAI ablation is planned well in advance and no thyroid hormone replacement is required in the interim period to allow TSH to rise.
- If the period between thyroidectomy and RAI ablation is longer, patients should stop liothyronine (T3) for 2 weeks or levothyroxine (T4) for 4 weeks before I^{131} ablation or therapy.
- Human recombinant TSH (Thyrogen™) 0.9 mg given intramuscularly on two consecutive days prior to I^{131} administration may be used without thyroid hormone withdrawal (THW) to avoid hypothyroid symptoms.
- Pregnancy must be excluded before I^{131} administration.
- Breast-feeding must be discontinued at least 4 weeks prior to I^{131} administration. Cabergoline may be used to stop lactation in selected cases.
- Pretreatment sperm storage should be considered in male patient who is likely to require repeat doses of radioiodine.

Radioiodine Remnant Ablation

- On the day of RAI ablation, check serum TSH, Tg levels, and renal function.
- TSH needs to be >30 mU/L at the time of I^{131} administration.
- The usual recommended I^{131} activity for RAI ablation is 3.7 GBq. However, recent prospective studies showed 1.1 Gbq provided equivalent ablation success rate as compared to 3.7 GBq in low-risk patients (Mallick et al. 2010; Catargi et al. 2010).
- In patients with known metastases, higher I^{131} activities (5–7.4 GBq) are often used.
- Patients need to be isolated until the whole body radioactivity comes down to a safe level prior to discharge depending on patients home circumstances.
- Post-ablation radioiodine scan should be performed 3–7 days after I^{131} administration. This would provide information on amount of thyroid remnant and distant metastasis.
- Start levothyroxine (T4) 3–4 days after I^{131} administration in patients who withdraw thyroid hormone prior to RAI. The usual adult dose is 150 mcg once a day.
- Advice to avoid pregnancy in female patients and fathering children in male patients for 4 months after I^{131} administration should be given.

Side Effects from Radioiodine Treatment

Early or short-term effects:

- Abnormal taste and sialadenitis (inflammation of parotid and submandibular glands). This may be minimized by good hydration during the period of isolation.
- Neck discomfort due to radioiodine induced thyroiditis when there is a large thyroid remnant present.
- Simple analgesic should be tried initially but a short course of steroids may be necessary for more severe cases.
- Nausea is possible and can be treated by antiemetics.
- Radiation induced cystitis and gastritis are not common.

Possible late effects:

- Salivary and lachrymal gland dysfunction may occur.
- Permanent dry mouth.
- Lifetime incidence of second cancers including leukemia is estimated to be around 0.5 %. The risk of leukemia is increased with a high cumulative dose of I^{131} >18.5 GBq.
- Infertility in both men and women especially with high cumulative doses.
- Radiation-induced pulmonary fibrosis may occur in patients with diffuse lung metastases following repeated doses of I^{131}.
- Increased risk of miscarriages may persist for up to a year after I^{131} administration.

Table 27.3 Risk categories for recurrent disease

Low risk	Intermediate risk	High risk
Complete macroscopic resection	Microscopic invasion of tumor in the extrathyroidal tissue	Macroscopic tumor invasion of local structures
No cervical lymph node metastasis (N0 disease)	N1 disease and cervical I^{131} uptake outside thyroid bed in the posttreatment I^{131} scan	Incomplete surgical resection
No distant metastasis	Tumor with aggressive histology or vascular invasion	Distant metastasis
No tumor invasion of locoregional structures		High Tg level out of proportion to what is seen on posttreatment I^{131} scan
No aggressive histology or vascular invasion		
No I^{131} uptake outside the thyroid bed in the posttreatment I^{131} scan		

Diagnostic Radioiodine Scans After RAI Ablation

- Diagnostic whole body I^{131} scans (WBS) are carried out to assess the effectiveness of the I^{131} ablation or therapy and the need for further investigation or treatment.
- The diagnostic WBS is usually carried out 8–12 months following RAI.
- The diagnostic WBS following recombinant human TSH (Thyrogen™) stimulation is preferable to THW to avoid hypothyroid symptoms.
- The preparation required for the diagnostic WBS with regard to low-iodine diet and THW or recombinant human TSH is the same as described above.
- TSH and Tg measurement should be done on the day of the diagnostic I^{131} WBS.
- TSH needs to be >30 mU/l at the time of WBS and Tg measurement.
- Undetectable Tg would suggest biochemically free of disease.
- Tg measurement following TSH stimulation and ultrasound neck without diagnostic I^{131} WBS in low-risk patient (see Table 27.3) is also an acceptable practice.

External Beam Radiotherapy (EBRT)

Adjuvant postoperative radiotherapy is infrequently indicated for DTC.
Indications for high-dose EBRT:

- Unresectable gross disease or cervical recurrent disease.
- Macroscopic residual disease following surgery.
- Microscopic residual disease following surgery where there is gross evidence of local tumor invasion and extensive extranodal spread.
- Residual tumor fails to concentrate sufficient amount of I^{131}.

Palliative radiotherapy is useful for:

- Painful bone metastasis
- Spinal cord compression
- Cerebral metastasis
- Symptomatic soft tissue or unresectable lymph node metastasis

Management of Hypocalcemia

- Serum calcium must be checked on the day after thyroidectomy.
- Hypocalcaemia should be treated with calcium supplementation. The usual starting dose of elemental calcium is 500 mg three times a day. The dose is adjusted according to response.
- Intravenous calcium gluconate may be necessary in some cases.
- Introduce calcitriol/alfacalcidol (vitamin D) if hypocalcaemia fails to improve. The usual dose of calcitriol to maintain normal calcium level is 0.5–2 μg a day.
- Hypoparathyroidism following total thyroidectomy is often transient and can be guided by parathyroid hormone (PTH) levels.
- In majority of cases, the calcitriol/alfacalcidol/calcium supplementation can be withdrawn on a gradual basis under close clinical supervision.

Risk Categorization

Three level of risk stratification for the assessment of the risk of recurrence (Table 27.3) recommended by the ATA (Cooper et al. 2009), which may be useful to determine the frequency of follow-up and the level of TSH suppression.

TSH Suppression

- DTC expresses TSH receptor on cell membrane and responds to TSH stimulation by increasing the rates of cell growth.
- Supraphysiologic doses of levothyroxine (T4) are used to suppress the TSH production in the effort to reduce the risk of recurrence.
- Long-term TSH suppression could be associated with increased risk of osteoporosis and cardiac arrhythmia.
- The level of TSH suppression in different risk categories recommended by ATA (Cooper et al. 2009) is summarized in Table 27.4.

Table 27.4 Level of TSH suppression recommended by ATA

Risk category	Level of TSH suppression
Low risk	
Biochemically and clinically free of disease	0.3–2 mU/L
Including patients who have not had RAI ablation	
Intermediate risk	
Biochemically and clinically free of disease	0.3–2 mU/L
High risk	
Persistent disease	<0.1 mU/L indefinitely
Biochemically and clinically free of disease	0.1–0.5 mU/L for 5–10 years

Measurement of Thyroglobulin During Follow-Up

- Thyroglobulin (Tg) is secreted by both normal thyroid follicular epithelium and cancerous thyroid cells.
- Patients who did not have RAI ablation following total thyroidectomy, the Tg measurement is limited by the inability to differentiate the source of Tg production between thyroid remnant and tumor.
- Rising Tg levels during follow-up on suppressive levothyroxine therapy is indicative of tumor recurrence or progression.
- 25 % of the population have thyroglobulin antibodies (Tg ab) which may or may not disappear following RAI ablation.
- The presence of Tg ab may cause interference in Tg assay. Neck ultrasonography is recommended for surveillance in patients with Tg ab.

Tips	Tricks
Patients are allowed <50 mcg iodine per day when on low-iodine diet	Many foods may contain small amount of iodine
Use recombinant human TSH for RAI ablation and diagnostic I[131] scan to avoid hypothyroid symptoms	Recombinant human TSH can be costly as compared to thyroid hormone withdrawal
Titrate levothyroxine dose based on thyroid function test and clinical symptoms	Assess the risk of recurrence and the level of TSH suppression required
Use clinical examination and neck ultrasound for surveillance in patients with thyroglobulin antibodies	Interference in thyroglobulin measurement in patients with thyroglobulin antibodies

References and Further Reading

British Thyroid Association, Royal College of Physicians London. Guidelines for the management of thyroid cancer. 2nd ed. London: British Thyroid Association and Royal College of Physicians; 2007.

Catargi B, Borget I, Deandreis D, Zerdoud S, Bridji B, Bardet S, Rousseau A, Bastie D, Schvartz C, Vera P, Morel O, Benisvy D, Bournaud C, Bonichon F, Dejax C, Toubert ME, Benhamou E,

Schlumberger M. Comparison of four strategies of radioiodine ablation in patients with thyroid cancer with low-risk of recurrence: the randomized, prospective ESTIMABL study on 753 patients. Paris: International Thyroid Congress; 2010. Abstract OC-067.

Cooper DS, Doherty GM, Haugen BR, Kloos RT, Lee SL, Mandel SJ, Mazzaferri EL, McIver B, Pacini F, Schlumberger M, Sherman SI, Steward DL, Tuttle RM. Revised American Thyroid Association management guidelines for patients with thyroid nodules and differentiated thyroid cancer. Thyroid. 2009;19(11):1167–214.

Kloos RT, Eng C, Evans DB, Francis GL, Gagel RF, Gharib H, Moley JF, Pacini F, Ringel MD, Schulumberger M, Wells SA. Medullary thyroid carcinoma: management guidelines of the American Thyroid Association. Thyroid. 2009;19(6):565–612.

Mallick U, Harmer C, Clarke S, Moss L, Nicol A, Clarke P, Smellie J, McCready R, Farnell K, Franklyn J, John R, Nutting C, Yap B, Lemon C, Wadlsey J, Gerrard G, Roques T, Macias E, Whitaker S, Abdul-Hamid A, Alvarez P, Kadalayil L, Hackshaw A. HiLo. Multicentre randomised phase III clinical trial of high versus low dose radioiodine, with or without recombinant human thyroid stimulating hormone (rhTSH), for remnant ablation for differentiated thyroid cancer. Paris: International Thyroid Congress; 2010. Abstract OC-068.

Pacini F, Schlumber M, Dralle H, Elisei R, Smit JWA, Wiersinga W, European Thyroid Cancer Taskforce. European consensus for the management of patients with differentiated thyroid carcinoma of the follicular epithelium. Eur J Endocrinol. 2008;154:787–803.

Chapter 28
Recent Advances in Thyroid Surgery

Joel Anthony Smith and Gregory P. Sadler

Introduction

The principles of thyroid surgery, meticulous anatomical dissection, careful vascular ligation, and preservation of surrounding structures, remain unchanged since they were popularized by Theodor Kocher in the late nineteenth century. The image of thyroid surgery has shifted away from the "horrible butchery" described by Gross in 1,866, to routine, same-day, or even outpatient surgery. In part this is due to technological advances along with a greater understanding of the anatomy and physiology of the gland. Recent advances in thyroid surgery can be divided into:

Improvements in clinical management and patient selection
Technology and equipment
Improvements in surgical safety

Although mortality is now rare in thyroid surgery, the focus in surgical technique has shifted to minimizing surgical morbidity and, more recently, improving surgical cosmesis.

Whatever techniques are employed to achieve this, it is well recognized that complications are minimized when thyroid surgery is carried out by dedicated, high-volume endocrine or head and neck surgeons:

J.A. Smith, FRCS (ORL-HNS), MBChB, BMedSc, DOHNS (✉)
Department of Otolaryngology, Head and Neck Surgery,
University Hospital Birmingham, Queen Elizabeth Medical Centre,
Edgbaston, Birmingham, West Midlands B15 2TH, UK
e-mail: joelsmith999@hotmail.com

G.P. Sadler, MD, FCRS Gen Surg (Eng)
Department of Endocrine Surgery, John Radcliffe Hospital,
Headley Way, Headington, Oxford, Oxon OX3 9DU, UK

J.C. Watkinson, D.M. Scott-Coombes (eds.), *Tips and Tricks in Endocrine Surgery*,
DOI 10.1007/978-1-4471-2146-6_28, © Springer-Verlag London 2014

Mortality occurs most commonly from bleeding in the neck and the resultant airway compromise.

Morbidity most often occurs due to injury to the laryngeal nerves (superior and recurrent) and parathyroid glands

Both are significant sources of litigation.

Advances in Clinical Management and Patient Selection

Who Should Perform Thyroid Surgery?

High-volume practice is likely to minimize complications and improves patient outcomes. Although most thyroid surgery is routine, difficult cases such as retrosternal or recurrent goiter and malignancy can cause significant challenges. Identification of the difficult case is the key to minimizing risk in thyroid surgery and is likely to be best achieved by high-volume surgeons. As well as high-volume practice thyroid surgeons should:

Be affiliated to national surgical associations.

Continuously audit their own practice.

Submit their data for national audit and comparison (as recommended by the British Association of Thyroid and Endocrine Surgeons (BAETS)).

This model of surgical practice is likely to become standard in the UK and around the world.

Advances in Diagnostics

Accuracy of patient selection defines when to and more importantly when not to operate. Cytological as well as radiological assessment of the thyroid gland have improved, giving more prognostic information and aiding in both decision making and surgical planning. These improvements decrease unnecessary surgery, lead to more appropriate first-time surgery, and are recommended by the American Thyroid Association in the assessment of all nodular disease. Risk stratification in nodular thyroid disease has improved due to:

More cytopathologists and radiologists with special interest in thyroid disease

Improvements in cytological grading systems that allow greater comparison of data between units

Greater yield from fine needle aspiration cytology (FNAC) with ultrasound guidance

Presentation of cytology and histology in multidisciplinary meetings

Improved assessment of thyroid nodules discovered incidentally

Technology and Equipment

Minimal Access Neck Surgery

Throughout surgical practice there has been a move towards decreasing the size of the access incision and its corresponding morbidity. The case for minimal access surgery has been made in abdominal and thoracic surgery due to major benefits in patient mobilization and recovery. Thyroid surgery differs in several important ways:

> Many procedures are carried out on a 23-h basis with limited morbidity associated with the standard surgical incision.
> Mobilization is good with standard access surgery.
> Pain is often not a major issue.

Cosmesis, however, is an important issue for some patients undergoing thyroid surgery due to the position and visibility of the wound. Studies suggest that in selected patients postoperative pain and cosmetic appearance may be improved using minimal access techniques. This is particularly important in certain ethnic groups and those prone to keloid formation. Much of the drive and innovation has come from Korea and Japan where acceptability of neck scars in women is lower. Cosmetic issues must be balanced against the often high costs and significant increases in operative time associated with minimal access techniques.

Several well-described techniques exist including minimal access neck surgery, endoscopic/visual assisted thyroid surgery (VATS), and transaxillary robotic surgery. Both minimal access and robotic surgery aim to either decrease the size of the neck wound or place incisions distant from the neck in cosmetically more acceptable positions. Figs. 28.1, 28.2, and 28.3 show typical minimal access surgical incisions.

Robotic Surgery

The use of robotic systems when operating on the thyroid gland has been developed in South Korea using the da Vinci three- or four-arm robot. There are now series of up 1,000 cases in the published literature and likely to be many more in the future as access to robotic surgery increases. Some argue the robot is better suited to the relatively confined space within the neck than laparoscopic instruments and, using specially designed retractors, has overcome many of the challenges in developing distant access surgery. Its use is being increased in North America and Europe. Surgical incisions are placed in the axilla, obviating the need for a neck incision (Fig. 28.4). There are no additional benefits to this approach however and wound morbidity may be increased due to the greater amount of dissection required as well as potential paresthesia to the upper chest.

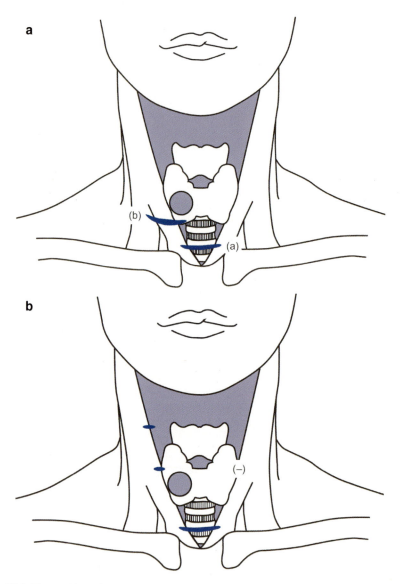

Fig. 28.1 The position of the incisions. (**a**) One 2 cm incision is made 1 cm above the sternal notch (*a*) or close to the position of the tumor (*b*). (**b**) The main transverse incision is made at the suprasternal notch and other incisions at the anterior margin of the sternomastoid muscle (Reproduced with permission from Shimizu K. Minimally invasive thyroid surgery. In: Best practice & research clinical endocrinology and metabolism, vol. 15, No. 2. Elsevier; 2001. p. 123–37)

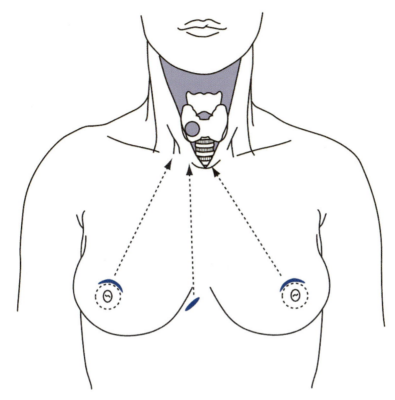

Fig. 28.2 Incisions along the mammary areola and at the parasternal site approaching the thyroid, indicated by *dotted lines*. The working space is created by carbon dioxide insufflation (Reproduced with permission from Shimizu K. Minimally invasive thyroid surgery. In: Best practice & research clinical endocrinology and metabolism, vol. 15, No. 2. Elsevier; 2001. p. 123–37)

In both minimal access and robotic surgery:

Access should not impair the surgical objectives.
Care should be taken with patient selection, particularly in obese patients or those advanced cancers or retro sternal goiter.
A consideration of additional costs should be made.
There may be increased length of hospital stay secondary to prolonged general anesthesia.

Surgical Equipment

Reducing bleeding intraoperatively and postoperatively has been a desirable objective and leads to a number of advances in all surgical fields. Much of the advancement has come from laparoscopic technology. There is increasing use in thyroid surgery of devices that coagulate and cut simultaneously including ultrasonic or

Fig. 28.3 Incisions at the axillary area. Three trocars and operative equipment are inserted through the wounds. The working space is obtained by carbon dioxide insufflation (Reproduced with permission from Shimizu K. Minimally invasive thyroid surgery. In: Best practice & research clinical endocrinology and metabolism, vol. 15, No. 2. Elsevier; 2001. p. 123–37)

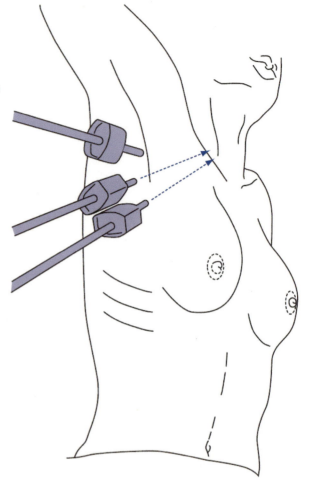

harmonic scalpels and bipolar cutting devices. In some centers these devices have superseded traditional ligatures or diathermy techniques and are particular benefi-cial if access is limited, for example, when ligating the upper pole. Charring is mini-mal and the degree of heat transferred to lateral tissues is reduced. This has advantages when operating close to the laryngeal nerves and parathyroid glands. Use of the harmonic scalpel has been linked to significantly decreased surgical time as well as improved postoperative pain. Many also advocate the use of these devices to reduce operative time allow the surgeon to approach more challenging parts of the operation with less fatigue.

Fig. 28.4 Robotic
thyroidectomy by a gasless
unilateral axillobreast
approach. (**a**) A 5–6-cm skin
incision was made in the
axillary fossa and a 0.8-cm
incision was made on the
circumareolar margin. (**b**) An
external retractor was used to
maintain the working space
without CO_2 gas insufflation.
In the axillary port, an
endoscope was placed in the
center and two robotic arms
were placed on either side of
the endoscope. The fourth
arm of the da Vinci S robot
was placed through the breast
port for retraction of the
thyroid gland with Prograsp.
(**c**) The view after placement
of the four robotic arms
(Reproduced with permission
from Tae K, et al. Robotic
thyroidectomy by a gasless
unilateral axillo-breast or
axillary approach: our early
experiences. Surg Endosc.
2011;25:221–8, Springer)

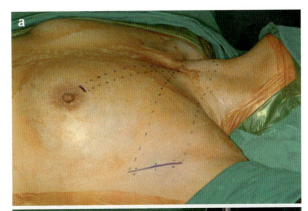

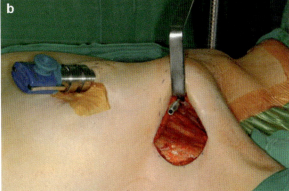

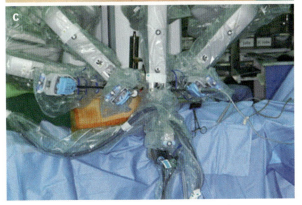

Surgical Safety

Calcium Optimization

Postoperative hypocalcemia in total thyroidectomy can lead to delayed discharge, the need for short- or long-term calcium replacement, or more serious complications such as tetany and cardiac arrhythmia. Postoperative hypocalcemia can be difficult to predict. As the half-life of parathyroid hormone (PTH) is much shorter than calcium, early PTH assay can predict those likely to need calcium replacement and also those suitable for early discharge. Endemic vitamin D deficiency is also an issue, particularly in migrant populations with darker skin living in regions with lower levels of sunlight. Some units advocate routine vitamin D assessment prior to thyroid surgery with calcium and vitamin replacement as needed to minimize the need for postoperative calcium supplementation.

Intraoperative Monitoring

Intraoperative recurrent laryngeal nerve (RLN) monitoring is now widely used. The most commonly used devices employ EMG monitoring mounted on a specially designed endotracheal tube and allow both monitoring and stimulation of the RLN. Monitoring devices however are not substitutes for anatomical knowledge and experience and should be used to confirm the position of the nerve rather than to search for it. Studies suggest no significant difference in rates of RLN palsy when comparing monitored and non-monitored groups. Most surgeons who use nerve monitors recommend doing so at all times such that when it is really useful such as in a difficult case, the theater team are familiar with the device.

Operative Checklists

Recently the World Health Organization (WHO) Checklist has been widely adopted and has been shown to be of benefit in healthcare systems across the world. Communication between health professionals lies at the heart of this. Focusing on pre- and postoperative patient medical optimization is likely to reduce complication such as DVT and cardiac anomalies and lead to better outcomes. With ageing populations and increasing medical complexity, these interventions are likely to become increasingly important.

Pearls and Pitfalls
Pearls

- If using technology such as nerve monitoring the surgical team should become familiar with the equipment during routine operations in order that it is of maximal benefit when a difficult case presents itself
- Surgeons should always rely on good judgement and sound anatomical knowledge
- Trainees should develop a wide range of experience with different technologies and not become too reliant on one particular device or technique

Pitfalls

- Redesigning a surgical procedure with a low morbidity and mortality will always be challenging
- New technologies often come with a learning curve which may lead to an unacceptable increase in morbidity
- Technological advances are often costly and may be difficult to justify where a clear case for improved morbidity or mortality cannot be made
- The availability of technology alone does not justify its use

Further Reading

British Thyroid Association Guidelines on the management of thyroid cancer. 2007. http://www.british-thyroid-association.org/news/Docs/Thyroid_cancer_guidelines_2007.pdf.   Accessed Jan 2011.

Cooper DS, Doherty GM, Haugen BR, Kloos RT, et al. Revised American Thyroid Association Guidelines for patients with thyroid nodules and differentiated thyroid cancer. Thyroid. 2009;19(11):1167–214.

Ecker T, Carvalho AL, Choe JH, Walosek G, et al. Hemostasis in thyroid surgery: harmonic scalpel versus other techniques—a meta-analysis. Otolaryngol Head Neck Surg. 2010;143:17–25.

Ferzli G, Sayaf P, Abdo Z, Cacchione R. Minimally invasive, nonendoscopic thyroid surgery. J Am Coll Surg. 2001;192(5):665–8.

Grodski S, Serpell J. Evidence for the role of perioperative PTH measurement after total thyroidectomy as a predictor of hypocalcemia. World J Surg. 2008;32(7):1367–73.

Higgins TS, Gupta R, Ketcham AS, Sataloff RT, Wadsworth JT, Sinacori JT. Recurrent laryngeal nerve monitoring versus identification alone on post-thyroidectomy true vocal fold palsy: a meta-analysis. Laryngoscope. 2011;121(5):1009–17.

Kang SW, Park JH, Jeong JS, Lee CR, et al. Prospects of robotic thyroidectomy using a gasless, transaxillary approach for the management of thyroid carcinoma. Surg Laparosc Endosc Percutan Tech. 2011;21(4):223–9.

Maeda S, Shimizu K, Minami S, Hayashida N, et al. Video-assisted neck surgery for thyroid and parathyroid diseases. Biomed Pharmacother. 2002;56(1):92–5.

Safe surgery saves lives. World Health Organisation. 2008. http://www.who.int/patientsafety/safe-surgery/en/. Accessed Jan 2011.

Smith JA, Watkinson JC, Shaha A. Who should perform thyroid surgery? United Kingdom (UK) and United States (US) perspectives with recommendations. Eur Arch Otorhinolaryngol. 2011; 269(1):1–4.

Sywak A, Yeh M, McMullen T, Stalberg P, et al. A randomized controlled trial of minimally invasive thyroidectomy using the lateral direct approach versus conventional hemithyroidectomy. Surgery. 2008;144(6):1016–22.

Tae K, Ji YB, Jeong JH, Lee S, et al. Robotic thyroidectomy by a gasless unilateral axillo-breast or axillary approach: our early experiences. Surg Endosc. 2011;25:221–8.

Yao HS, Wang Q, Wang WJ, Ruan CP. Prospective clinical trials of thyroidectomy with ligaSure vs conventional vessel ligation: a systematic review and meta-analysis. Arch Surg. 2009;144(12): 1167–74.

Chapter 29
Outcomes and Audit in Endocrine Surgery

Richard Wight and David M. Scott-Coombes

Introduction

Clinical audit should be an integral part of all practicing surgeons' activities. To support audit in surgery, consideration is made of what makes a good audit and the steps needed to undertake it – finding and setting standards, data collection, analysis and interpretation, and action on audit results.

Why Audit Outcomes?

- To comply with Good Medical Practice – practitioners should take part in regular and systematic audit.
- Meeting Good Surgical Practice – surgeons should be aware of their results in their surgical practice.
- Surgeons should audit benchmark and share their results with peer groups and seek advice if there is a major discrepancy in their performance.
- Contribute in resolving uncertainties about the effects of treatments.

Audit should not be confused with research. For audit the outcomes (whether qualitative or quantitative) are measured against a defined standard.

R. Wight (✉)
Department of Otolaryngology, Head and Neck Surgery,
James Cook University Hospital,
Marton Road, Middlesbrough, UK
e-mail: richard.wight@stees.nhs.uk

D.M. Scott-Coombes, MS, FRCS
Department of Endocrine Surgery,
University Hospital of Wales, Heath Park,
Cardiff CF14 4XW, UK
e-mail: david.scott-coombes@wales.nhs.uk

J.C. Watkinson, D.M. Scott-Coombes (eds.), *Tips and Tricks in Endocrine Surgery*,
DOI 10.1007/978-1-4471-2146-6_29, © Springer-Verlag London 2014

What Makes a Good Audit?

- Prior careful consideration of an aspect(s) of surgery that is measurable and in which a change/improvement in practice will be beneficial.
- Formulating a question(s) as simply as possible to aid clarification to others.
- Deliverable within available resources (people, time, IT).
- In gaining local support, an alignment with an organization's audit priorities and early registration with the hospital clinical audit department can pay dividends both in help and quality.
- Contributing to national audit has the significant benefits of peer-to-peer comparisons so that local activity can concentrate on high-quality data submission and action arising from the findings.

  - Pre-provision of a collection modality/dataset
  - Receipt of analyzed outcomes

Finding and Setting the Standard(s)

- In establishing standards, a number of national reference sources/guidelines are available, e.g., Guidelines for the management of thyroid cancer 2007 British Thyroid Association, British Association of Endocrine and Thyroid Surgeons (BAETS), British Association of Head and Neck Oncology standards, and Royal College of Pathology reporting standards which may match to the topic under consideration.
- Consider standards used by peers.
- Having agreed a standard, define a baseline or criteria with the minimum expected level of performance, noting that setting 100 % as a criterion means it will rarely be achieved.
- A target for improvement can also be defined.

Collecting the Data

- Source data from existing collected sources to keep "new collection" to a minimum.
- Be clear about the methodology before designing a simple data collection proforma/tool.
- Decide about the methodology:

  - Retrospective or prospective
  - Time frame
  - Exclusion an inclusion criteria

- Collect the minimum amount of data to answer the audit question. Avoid straying into additional "wouldn't it be interesting" information.

- Discuss with colleagues to avoid pitfalls in missed information.
- At the outset consider a pilot study.
- Make sure collection/storage is compatible with local information governance procedures particularly in relation to patient confidentiality/data protection law.

Analysis and Interpretation

- Seek statistical help if needed prior to starting data collection.
- Understand the range of variation – has the standard been reached? Has the target for improvement been met; if not, what may be the contributory factors?
- Apply appropriate statistical tests depending on the nature of the variable being studied.
- Present data in a range of visual formats to improve understanding.

Actions from Findings

- To support implementation of change and propose an action plan.
- In the action plan identify who, what, and in what time frame is suggested.
- Are new or different resources needed?
- Share your findings with others.
- Having implemented the change, revisit the standards and agree the next cycle of audit.

Publication

There are a variety of audiences to whom audit may be of interest.

- Peers: to drive a change for improved practice
- Commissioners: to assist them in making decisions about funding
- Patients: to assist in making informed decisions about their care
- The public: to increase transparency

Specialist Society/National Audit

- BAETS has an audit of endocrine procedures. Members are able to submit to an online audit with the focus having been on short-term comorbidities, but now recent inclusion of standards (e.g., pre- and postoperative assessment of vocal cord movement).
- The National Cancer Intelligence Network has commenced work on developing proposals for national audit in thyroid cancer with a variety of stakeholders via a working group expected to report at the end of 2012.

Pearls and Pitfalls
Pearls in Clinical Audit

- Choose a topic that will produce change and benefit patient care
- Keep the question(s) simple
- Seek help early in the process from local clinical audit departments and register the audit with them
- Undertake a pilot to identify any gaps in data collection
- Present the findings in clear visual formats to engage others and influence successful change/improvement
- Contribute to national audit

Pitfalls in Clinical Audit

- Failing to contribute to local or national audit – revalidation is upon us!
- Confusing with research
- Not having defined standards to benchmark against
- Being over ambitious and failing to complete the audit cycle
- Overburdening data collection
- Presenting lots of data but little information
- Not acting on the findings

Further Reading

An introduction to statistics for clinical audit. HQIP. 2011. http://www.hqip.org.uk/assets/LQIT-uploads/Guidance-0112/HQIP-CA-PD-002-251111-An-Introduction-to-Statistics-for-Clinical-Audit.pdf.

British Association of Endocrine and Thyroid Surgeons. http://www.baets.org.uk/Pages/audit.php.

British Association of Head and Neck Oncologists Standards. 2009. http://www.bahno.org.uk/docs/BAHNO%20STANDARDS%20DOC09.pdf.

British Thyroid Association Guidelines and Statements. http://www.british-thyroid-association.org/Guidelines/.

Good Medical Practice. Maintaining good medical practice. General Medical Council. http://www.gmc-uk.org/guidance/good_medical_practice.asp.

Good Surgical Practice. Royal College of Surgeons of England. 2008 http://www.rcseng.ac.uk/publications/docs/good-surgical-practice-1.

National Cancer Intelligence Network. www.ncin.org.uk.

Standards and datasets for reporting cancers. Dataset for thyroid cancer histopathology reports. 2010. Royal College of Pathologists. http://www.rcpath.org/resources/pdf/g098datasetforthyroidcancerhistopathologyreportsfinal.pdf.

Chapter 30
Consent and Litigation in Thyroid Surgery

Barney Harrison

> *To err is human, to cover up is unforgivable and to fail to learn is inexcusable.*
>
> Sir Liam Donaldson, Chief Medical Officer for England 2004

Introduction

Prior to agreeing to a recommendation for thyroid surgery, the patient should be made aware of the indications for operation and its implications, risks, and potential complications. When the outcome from surgery is not as planned, be reassured that litigation after thyroidectomy is uncommon, and if appropriate decision-making took place before, during, and after operation, it is unlikely to succeed.

Consent

The consent process is a legal requirement prior to surgery; it requires the patient to have the capacity to understand the process and the nature and purpose of the operation. The patient should provide consent voluntarily.

As surgeons we should keep in mind that what we do does not always go the way we – and, more importantly, the patient – would wish. The inevitable companions in our professional life are "complications" – the undesirable, unintended, and direct result of surgery. Remember that complications may arise without errors as well as a result of errors, and errors can occur without associated complications.

B. Harrison, MBBS, MS, FRCS Eng
Department of Endocrine Surgery,
Royal Hallamshire Hospital, Glossop Road,
Sheffield S10 2JF, UK
e-mail: barney.harrison@sth.nhs.uk

J.C. Watkinson, D.M. Scott-Coombes (eds.), *Tips and Tricks in Endocrine Surgery*,   227
DOI 10.1007/978-1-4471-2146-6_30, © Springer-Verlag London 2014

When to Inform and Consent?

The patient should have time well in advance of the start of treatment to consider the information on risk and complications before they make a decision to proceed. There should be sufficient time between the discussion and the procedure taking place.

Who Should Do It?

Ideally, the doctor who undertakes the investigation or provides the treatment. If delegated, the person must be suitably trained and qualified and knowledgeable of the procedure.

What to Inform the Patient of?

Explain the indications for operation and the implications, risks, and complications in a way the patient can understand. If you have concerns with regard to the capacity of the patient to give consent, seek appropriate advice from other health-care professionals.

Diagrams and written information given to the patient are of benefit but not a substitute for adequate exchange of verbal information.

Significant risks should be disclosed that might affect the patient's judgement and decision-making, irrespective of the likelihood of their occurrence. In England and Wales, the numeric threshold is legally not relevant, except when treatments are being compared (Wheeler 2012).

Remember that thyroid surgery associated with a higher risk of postoperative bleeding, hypoparathyroidism, and recurrent laryngeal nerve palsy includes:

Retrosternal goiter
Thyroid cancer
Thyroid disease in children
Thyrotoxicosis
Reoperation
Thyroidectomy performed by low-volume surgeons
Thyroidectomy performed in low-volume hospitals

In terms of lowering risk, note that the only randomized study comparing intraoperative monitoring of the recurrent laryngeal nerve with nerve visualization alone did not show a reduction in the risk of permanent recurrent laryngeal palsy (Barczynski et al. 2009), and a recent retrospective study of patients undergoing reoperative thyroid surgery with and without the nerve monitor failed to show a benefit from nerve monitoring (Alesina et al. 2012).

Remember that a signed consent form in the clinical records may not be enough to demonstrate informed consent.

The patients' notes should record information discussed with the patient – including the specific risks and complications, details of written or other information given to the patient, and details of the decisions made.

Litigation

Facts

In 2010/2011 the National Health Service Litigation Authority received 8,655 claims under its clinical negligence scheme. Payments made in the financial year 2010/2011 for clinical negligence were over £863 million. Compare that with the USA where the annual costs associated with medical liability – including legal costs and payouts, malpractice insurance, and the practice of defensive medicine – are £36.2 billion (Mello et al. 2010).

Fewer than 50 clinical negligence cases a year are contested in court; the outcomes of medical negligence claims against the NHS from April 2001 to March 2011 were as follows:

Abandoned by client	37.7 %
Settled out of court	45 %
Damages approved by court	3.16 %
Yet to settle	14.14 %

Definitions

Duty of care is the watchfulness, attention, caution, and prudence that a reasonable person in the circumstances would exercise. A breach of duty is when the care given is below the standard the patient had a right to expect and injury occurs.

Causation is the establishment of a link between the breach of duty and the injuries complained of.

What Information Is Available with Regard to the Frequency of Litigation After Thyroid Surgery?

From the USA it is reported that the rate of post-thyroidectomy malpractice claims is 5.9 per 10,000 cases (Singer et al. 2012). Eighty-nine percent of cases occur after routine thyroid surgery, deficient informed consent is the issue in 11 % (Lydiatt 2003), and 46 % of cases involve injury to the recurrent laryngeal nerve (Abadin et al. 2010). A review of claims specifically related to iatrogenic vocal cord palsy reported that 30 % occurred after thyroid/parathyroid surgery, in 36 % there was a failure to recognize the complication, and 19 % were consent issues (Shaw and Pierce 2009).

Claims following surgical injury to accessory nerve injury result from cervical lymph node biopsies (68 %) and neck dissections (5 %). Claim allegations include negligent surgical technique (98 %), lack of informed consent (21 %), and failure to diagnose the injury (20 %) (Morris et al. 2008).

In the UK there is little specific information on post-thyroidectomy litigation, but the National Health Service Litigation Authority recorded 17 claims involving thyroid surgery and damage to the vocal cords between 1995 and 2005 (Mihai and Randolph 2009).

Factors reported to increase the likelihood of a successful litigation claim after thyroid surgery include the need for a second operation, if the primary goal of an operation had been missed, and a complication is followed by a fault in postoperative care (Schulte and Roher 1999).

Expert Witness

Before you take on the role of an expert witness, you should be familiar with the relevant GMC guidance on your role and duties including knowledge of Civil Procedure rule 35.3.

Key issues that you must consider include the remit that the expert:

Represents a reasonable body of opinion
Gives a balanced opinion and is able to state the facts or assumptions on which it is based
Acts independently and is not influenced by the party that retains you
Does not omit material facts which could detract from his/her concluded opinion
Makes it clear when a particular question or issue falls outside his/her expertise
Is aware of the standards and nature of practice at the time of the incident under proceedings

Remember that the expert witness is no longer immune from actions of breach of duty that includes preparation of reports for service on the opposition, legal conferences, and oral evidence impartially.

Pearls and Pitfalls
Pearls
It goes better when you:

- Know your medicine.
- Warn of risks.
- Write accurate, detailed, legible notes.
- Do not believe what others tell you – find out for yourself.
- Identify early signs of a problem.
- Act promptly.

- Seek help early.
- Chase results that you order.
- Understand results that you order.

Ask yourself:

- Is the operation appropriate/necessary?
- Are you appropriately trained?
- Are you "up-to-date"?

Pitfalls

It goes wrong when there has been a failure to:

- Examine the patient properly.
- Diagnose.
- Inform the patient of the implications to have or not have the procedure.
- Give appropriate advice.
- Refer to an appropriate specialist.
- Operate competently.
- Interpret tests correctly/monitor/follow-up.

It gets worse because of:

- Inaction
- Lack of knowledge
- Failure to gather adequate data
- Misinterpretation of data
- Deficiencies in pre-/peri-/postoperative care

References

Abadin SS, Kaplan EL, Angelos P. Malpractice litigation after thyroid surgery: the role of recurrent laryngeal nerve injuries, 1989–2009. Surgery. 2010;148(4):718–22; discussion 22–3.

Alesina PF, Rolfs T, Hommeltenberg S, Hinrichs J, Meier B, Mohmand W, et al. Intraoperative neuromonitoring does not reduce the incidence of recurrent laryngeal nerve palsy in thyroid reoperations: results of a retrospective comparative analysis. World J Surg. 2012;36(6): 1348–53.

Barczynski M, Konturek A, Cichon S. Randomized clinical trial of visualization versus neuromonitoring of recurrent laryngeal nerves during thyroidectomy. Br J Surg. 2009;96(3):240–6.

Lydiatt DD. Medical malpractice and the thyroid gland. Head Neck. 2003;25(6):429–31.

Mello MM, Chandra A, Gawande AA, Studdert DM. National costs of the medical liability system. Health Aff (Millwood). 2010;29(9):1569–77.

Mihai R, Randolph G. Thyroid surgery, voice and the laryngeal examination—time for increased awareness and accurate evaluation. World J Endocr Surg. 2009;1:1.

Morris LG, Ziff DJ, Delacure MD. Malpractice litigation after surgical injury of the spinal accessory nerve: an evidence-based analysis. Arch Otolaryngol Head Neck Surg. 2008;134(1):102–7.

Schulte KM, Roher HD. Medico-legal aspects of thyroid surgery. Chirurg. 1999;70(10):1131–8.

Shaw GY, Pierce E. Malpractice litigation involving iatrogenic surgical vocal fold paralysis: a closed-claims review with recommendations for prevention and management. Ann Otol Rhinol Laryngol. 2009;118(1):6–12.

Singer MC, Iverson KC, Terris DJ. Thyroidectomy-related malpractice claims. Otolaryngol Head Neck Surg. 2012;146(3):358–61.

Wheeler R. The numeric threshold for the disclosure of risk: outdated and inapplicable to surgical consent. Ann R Coll Surg Engl. 2012;94(2):81–2.

Further Reading

Acting as an expert witness – Guidance for doctors. www.gmc-uk.org/guidance/ethical_guidance/expert_witness_guidance.asp.

Sokol DK. How can I avoid being sued? BMJ. 2011;343:d7827.

Part IV
Parathyroid

Chapter 31
Assessment of Hyperparathyroidism

Judit Konya, Mo Aye, R. James England, and Stephen L. Atkin

Abbreviations

BMD	Bone mineral density
CaE	Fractional excretion of calcium
CaHPO$_4$	Calcium phosphate
CaSR	Calcium-sensing receptor
dRTA	Distal renal tubular acidosis
FHH	Familial hypocalciuric hypercalcemia
MEN	Multiple endocrine neoplasia
PHPT	Primary hyperparathyroidism
PTA	Proximal renal tubular acidosis
PTH	Parathyroid hormone
PTHrP	Parathormone-related peptide

J. Konya, MBBS • S.L. Atkin, MBBS, FRCP, PhD (✉)
Department of Diabetes, Endocrinology and Metabolism,
University of Hull, Brocklehurst Building, Hull Royal Infirmary,
220-236 Anlaby Road, Hull, HU3 2RW, UK
e-mail: stephen.atkin@hyms.ac.uk; s.l.atkin@hull.ac.uk

M. Aye, MBBS, FRCP, FRCPEdin
Department of Diabetes, Endocrinology and Metabolism,
Centre for Metabolic Bone Disease Hull and East Yorkshire Hospitals NHS Trust,
Hull Royal Infirmary, Hull, UK

R.J. England, MBCHB, FRCS (ORL-HNS)
Department of ENT/Head and Neck Surgery, Hull and East Yorkshire Hospitals NHS Trust,
Castle Hill Hospital, Castle Street, Cottingham, Hull, East Riding of Yorkshire HU16 5JQ, UK

J.C. Watkinson, D.M. Scott-Coombes (eds.), *Tips and Tricks in Endocrine Surgery*,
DOI 10.1007/978-1-4471-2146-6_31, © Springer-Verlag London 2014

Background: Physiology

The cell surface of each parathyroid cell has a calcium-sensing receptor. The four parathyroid glands secrete parathyroid hormone (PTH). A fall in serum calcium stimulates the secretion of PTH that results in increase of the level of circulatory ionized calcium.

Skeletal Actions of PTH (Talmage and Elliott 1958)

- Immediate: mobilization of readily available calcium from skeletal stores that are in equilibrium with the extracellular fluid
- Delayed: activation of bone resorption leading to more calcium and phosphate release

Renal Actions of PTH (Broadus et al. 1980; Friedman and Gesek 1993; Pfister et al. 1997)

- Reabsorption of calcium
- Decreased reabsorption of phosphate
- Synthesis of calcitriol

Overall Actions of PTH

- Elevation of serum calcium
- Phosphaturia
- Calcitriol synthesis

Vitamin D3

The other principle hormone that affects plasma calcium is 1,25-dihydroxyvitamin D3 (calcitriol), the active metabolite of vitamin D. With PTH, calcitriol acts on the small intestine to increase calcium absorption. In opposition to PTH, calcitriol acts on the skeletal system and the kidneys (decrease of calcium and phosphate excretion) (Fig. 31.1).

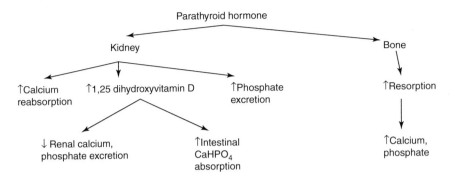

Fig. 31.1 Calcium homeostasis – the role of PTH and 1,25-dihydroxyvitamin D

Classification of Hyperparathyroidism

Primary

- Autonomous PTH secretion (single adenoma in 80–90 %, hyperplasia in 10–15 %, double adenoma in 2 %, and carcinoma <1 %), characterized by elevated serum calcium and PTH.

  Primary hyperparathyroidism (PHPT):

  - The third most common endocrinological disease, present in up to 1 in 500 of the general population where it is predominantly a disease of postmenopausal women.
  - The prevalence of PHPT in women less than 40 years old is 10/100,000 and 190/100,000 in women over 65 years of age.

  Multiple endocrine neoplasia (MEN) should be considered when a patient presents with PHPT below the age of 40 years with a family history of HPT.

  A recently recognized variant of the disease is normocalcemic PHPT (Tordjman et al. 2004) where the level of PTH is elevated but the calcium level is normal or close to the upper limit of the normal range. It has yet to be determined if this form of PHPT is a precursor of hypercalcemic PHPT or a unique phenotype of PHPT. Patients with normocalcemic PHPT are usually identified during an investigation based on low bone mineral density.

Secondary

- An appropriate physiological response to hypocalcemia characterized by elevated PTH and normal or low serum calcium concentrations.

Underlying possible causes of secondary hyperparathyroidism:

- Gastrointestinal disorder (malabsorption)
- Dietary vitamin D deficiency
- Synthetic vitamin D deficiency secondary to renal insufficiency (also known as renal HPT)
- Drugs (e.g., lithium, thiazides)

Tertiary

- This is unique to patients who have undergone a successful renal transplantation. Rarely post transplantation (2 %), the preexisting secondary (renal) HPT develops into an inappropriate autonomous hypersecretion of PTH (akin to PHPT) resulting in hypercalcemia.

Clinical Manifestations

PHPT is most commonly associated with minimally symptomatic hypercalcemia that may be increasingly identified through the use of laboratory biochemical profiles that include calcium measurement (Silverberg and Bilezikian 1996).

The clinical manifestations of hyperparathyroidism are based on the effects of excess serum calcium. Elderly people are more sensitive to the symptoms even at lower levels of hypercalcemia. The classical signs and symptoms of hypercalcemia are much less commonly seen but include (Inzucchi 2004):

The effects of an increased level of PTH include (Bilezikian et al. 2005):

- Signs and symptoms of hypercalcemia (Table 31.1).
- Parathyroid bone disease.

  - Decreased bone mineral density (BMD), particularly in cortical bone rather than cancellous bone
  - Osteitis fibrosa cystica (rarely seen but includes):

    - Bone pain
    - Subperiosteal bone resorption (middle phalanges radial aspect)
    - Distal clavicular tapering
    - "Salt and pepper" appearance of the skull
    - Bone cysts
    - Brown tumors of the bones

- Renal manifestations:
Decreased urinary concentrating ability leading to hypophosphatemia and hypomagnesemia

Table 31.1 Manifestations of hypercalcemia

Renal manifestations: polyuria and polydipsia due to hypercalciuria and the decreased
  concentration capacity of the kidneys; nephrocalcinosis and/or nephrolithiasis; dRTA; renal
  insufficiency
Gastrointestinal manifestations: nausea, decreased appetite, vomiting, obstipation, peptic ulcer,
  pancreatitis
Other manifestations: fatigue, confusion, coma, musculoskeletal pain, decreased muscle
  strength, osteopenia or osteoporosis, hypertension, abnormal ECG findings (bradycardia,
  QT shortening)

Nephrolithiasis (mainly calcium oxalate stones) and nephrocalcinosis
Proximal renal tubular acidosis (PTA)
- Increased calcitriol level.
- Hyperuricemia and gout.
- Anemia: due to severe PHPT.
- Cardiovascular diseases (Andersson et al. 2004): PHPT may be associated with hypertension, left ventricular hypertrophy and diastolic dysfunction, and increased vessel stiffness. It has also been suggested that vessel stiffness may be related to the severity of hyperparathyroidism.

Diagnosis and Differential Diagnosis of PHPT

Primary hyperparathyroidism is usually first suspected due to an elevated calcium concentration found as an incidental finding or through investigation of the symptoms of hypercalcemia.

Serum calcium (corrected to serum albumin) should be repeated, and previous calcium results should be reviewed, if available, to look for long-term asymptomatic hypercalcemia.

In 80–90 % of the patients with PHPT, there is an elevated serum concentration of PTH; however, 10–20 % of the patients have a PTH either mildly elevated or within the normal range (Nussbaum et al. 1987).

PHPT can be confirmed with the findings of:

- Hypercalcemia (on two serum calcium measurements)
- PTH elevated (or inappropriately at high end of reference range in the face of hypercalcemia)
- No lithium or thiazide therapy
- Urinary calcium to creatinine >0.01

In patients with PHPT, neck examination is usually unrevealing as adenomas are usually not palpable.

If a neck mass is present in association with severe PHPT, consider parathyroid carcinoma.

Bone mineral density is not necessary to confirm the diagnosis, but decreased bone mineral density may influence whether surgery is undertaken.

Localization studies should not be undertaken to determine the diagnosis, but may be of value if minimally invasive surgery is considered.

Malignancy

- PHPT is the commonest cause of hypercalcemia, followed by malignancy.
- In most cases malignancy is clinically evident and is associated with an elevated calcium level and undetectable PTH levels.
- Hypercalcemia of malignancy is mainly due to ectopic hormone production with secretion of parathormone-related peptide (PTHrP) (80 %). The biochemical assays for PTH and PTHrP are distinct. The remainder is usually due to osteolysis from extensive bone metastases (Stewart 2005).

Familial Hypocalciuric Hypercalcemia (FHH)

- This is a very rare autosomal dominant inherited condition due to an inactivating mutation of the calcium-sensing receptor resulting in a "resetting" of the normal range for serum calcium. This results in PTH levels that become normal only in the presence of increased calcium levels (Fuleihan Gel 2002).
- The hypercalcemia does not cause symptoms and does not require treatment.
- It may be difficult to differentiate between FHH and PHPT, but this can be resolved by calculating the Ca/Cr clearance ratio.
  That is, the fractional excretion of calcium (CaE): PHPT CaE $\geq$200, FHH CaE <100.

$$CaE = \frac{24-h \text{ urine calcium}\,(mmol)}{24-h \text{ urine creatinine}\,(micromol)} \times \frac{plasma \text{ creatinine}\,(micromol)}{plasma \text{ calcium}\,(mmol)}$$

- When there is a strong clinical suspicion of FHH, patients can be tested for the specific genetic mutation.

Drugs

- Lithium decreases parathyroid gland sensitivity to calcium and reduces urinary calcium excretion (Mallette et al. 1989).
- Thiazide diuretics cause reduced urinary calcium excretion alone (Christensson et al. 1977).

Management of Hyperparathyroidism

In patients with symptomatic PHPT, parathyroidectomy is the preferred treatment option.

In accord with the Third International Workshop guidelines (Bilezikian et al. 2009), surgery is indicated in asymptomatic patients who meet any of the following:

- Serum calcium concentration of 1.0 mg/dL (0.25 mmol/L) or more above the upper limit of normal.
- Creatinine clearance reduced to <60 mL/min.
- Bone density at the hip, lumbar spine, and distal radius is more than 2.5 standard deviations below peak bone mass (T score <−2.5) and/or previous fragility fracture.
- Age less than 50 years.

In asymptomatic patients over the age of 50 then monitoring alone may be appropriate and may include:

1. Prevention:
   - Avoid factors that can cause hypercalcemia (i.e., drug therapy, a high calcium diet, prolonged bed rest).
   - Encourage physical activity and adequate hydration.
   - Maintain moderate Ca (1,000 mg/day) and vitamin D intake (400–600 IU/day).

2. Monitoring:
   - Serum calcium and creatinine annually
   - BMD every second year

3. Medication:
   - Bisphosphonates are useful for treatment of osteoporosis.

- Concomitant vitamin D deficiency should be carefully treated as supplementation of vitamin D may rise calciuria quickly and increases the risk of kidney stone formation.

In patients with secondary hyperparathyroidism, the therapy should focus on the treatment of the underlying medical condition.

Pearls and Pitfalls
Pearls

- Primary hyperparathyroidism is a common endocrinological disease, often found coincidently, where the definitive treatment is parathyroidectomy
- The clinical manifestations of PHPT are usually mild if present

Pitfalls

- Calcium measurement should be repeated in order to confirm diagnosis
- Calcium and parathyroid hormone levels should only be interpreted in the knowledge of the 1,25-dihydroxyvitamin D level
- The fractional excretion of calcium should be performed in young asymptomatic patients

---

References

Andersson P, Rydberg E, et al. Primary hyperparathyroidism and heart disease–a review. Eur Heart J. 2004;25(20):1776–87.

Bilezikian JP, Brandi ML, et al. Primary hyperparathyroidism: new concepts in clinical, densitometric and biochemical features. J Intern Med. 2005;257(1):6–17.

Bilezikian JP, Khan AA, et al. Guidelines for the management of asymptomatic primary hyperparathyroidism: summary statement from the third international workshop. J Clin Endocrinol Metab. 2009;94(2):335–9.

Broadus AE, Horst RL, et al. The importance of circulating 1,25-dihydroxyvitamin D in the pathogenesis of hypercalciuria and renal-stone formation in primary hyperparathyroidism. N Engl J Med. 1980;302(8):421–6.

Christensson T, Hellstrom K, et al. Hypercalcemia and primary hyperparathyroidism. Prevalence in patients receiving thiazides as detected in a health screen. Arch Intern Med. 1977;137(9): 1138–42.

Friedman PA, Gesek FA. Calcium transport in renal epithelial cells. Am J Physiol. 1993;264(2 Pt 2): F181–98.

Fuleihan Gel H. Familial benign hypocalciuric hypercalcemia. J Bone Miner Res. 2002;17 Suppl 2:N51–6.

Inzucchi SE. Understanding hypercalcemia. Its metabolic basis, signs, and symptoms. Postgrad Med. 2004;115(4):69–70. 73–6.

Mallette LE, Khouri K, et al. Lithium treatment increases intact and midregion parathyroid hormone and parathyroid volume. J Clin Endocrinol Metab. 1989;68(3):654–60.

Nussbaum SR, Zahradnik RJ, et al. Highly sensitive two-site immunoradiometric assay of parathyrin, and its clinical utility in evaluating patients with hypercalcemia. Clin Chem. 1987;33(8):1364–7.

Pfister MF, Lederer E, et al. Parathyroid hormone-dependent degradation of type II Na+/Pi cotrans-
    porters. J Biol Chem. 1997;272(32):20125–30.
Silverberg SJ, Bilezikian JP. Evaluation and management of primary hyperparathyroidism. J Clin
    Endocrinol Metab. 1996;81(6):2036–40.
Stewart AF. Clinical practice. Hypercalcemia associated with cancer. N Engl J Med. 2005;352(4):
    373–9.
Talmage RV, Elliott JR. Removal of calcium from bone as influenced by the parathyroids.
    Endocrinology. 1958;62(6):717–22.
Tordjman KM, Greenman Y, et al. Characterization of normocalcemic primary hyperparathyroid-
    ism. Am J Med. 2004;117(11):861–3.

Chapter 32
Parathyroidectomy: Indications for Surgery and Localization

Gregory P. Sadler

Indications for Surgery in Parathyroid Disease

Symptomatic Patients

All symptomatic patients with hyperparathyroidism (HPT) should be considered for surgery. Symptoms in HPT are often rather nonspecific, and it may be difficult to attribute any given symptom directly to the disease. Symptoms/presentation clearly in need of treatment includes:

- *Renal stones*
- *Osteoporosis*
- *Hypercalcemic crisis*

  Other less easily definable symptoms may include:

- *Tiredness/lethargy*
- *Muscular aches and pains, bone pain*
- *Polydipsia, polyuria, nocturia*
- *Difficulty concentrating, memory loss, mild confusion*
- *Abdominal cramps, constipation*

Asymptomatic Patients

Offering surgery for patients who are totally asymptomatic is a contentious issue. There has to be a clear demonstration of future health benefits versus the potential

G.P. Sadler, MD, FRCS Gen Surg (Eng)
Department of Endocrine Surgery, John Radcliffe Hospital,
Headley Way, Headington, Oxford OX3 9DU, UK
e-mail: gregsadler@btinternet.com

J.C. Watkinson, D.M. Scott-Coombes (eds.), *Tips and Tricks in Endocrine Surgery*,
DOI 10.1007/978-1-4471-2146-6_32, © Springer-Verlag London 2014

adverse outcome of surgery. There are several studies suggesting that very few patients are truly asymptomatic and that following curative surgery patients previously considered to be asymptomatic show improvement in Quality of Life Scores.

In 1990, the NIH issued a consensus statement on the management of patients with asymptomatic HPT. This guidance was updated in 2009. Parathyroid surgery in truly asymptomatic patients is recommended where:

- Age <50 years old
- Plasma calcium >0.25 mmol/l above normal range
- Urinary calcium excretion >10 mmol/day
- Creatinine clearance reduced by 30 %
- Bone mineral density (at any site) reduced by 2.5 standard deviations

Hypothetical Benefits of Surgery in Asymptomatic Patients

- Bone density improved (decreased chance of fracture a major cause of morbidity in elderly patients)
- Decreased incidence of cardiac morbidity and death
- Improved glucose and lipid metabolism

There is published evidence to support all the above points; however, this remains relatively weak, and many physicians would argue against the need for patients with mild (biochemical) hyperparathyroidism undergoing surgery.

Localization for First-Time Parathyroid Surgery

Important: Localization should not be used to confirm parathyroid disease and should be performed only after biochemical confirmation of HPT.

In the hands of an experienced parathyroid surgeon, cure rates above 95 % are achievable with an "open" bilateral cervical exploration through a midline incision, with no prior imaging studies.

Localization of parathyroid tumors is therefore not needed:

- In high-volume centers where the surgeon is experienced and happy to proceed without imaging studies
- Total or subtotal parathyroidectomy for renal hyperparathyroidism or multiple endocrine neoplasia (MEN) (imaging studies do not help)

Localization should be performed:

- Only following biochemical confirmation of the disease
- In low-volume centers (if this is thought likely to increase the success of the procedure)
- Where minimally invasive parathyroidectomy (MIP) is contemplated
- In all cases of reoperative surgery

Elective First-Time Surgery Primary HPT

- Preoperative localization studies are not needed for parathyroid surgery in experienced hands.
- Advocates of routine pre-op localization for all patients would argue that when positive:
  - Operative time can be planned more accurately
  - Procedures are shortened
  - Potential to demonstrate ectopic glands in the chest thus avoiding unnecessary and lengthy negative cervical exploration
- Accurate, preoperative localization of a likely benign solitary parathyroid tumor is clearly required if MIP is considered appropriate for the patient.
- In patients where intraoperative PTH (ioPTH) estimation is not used perioperatively, increased cure rate is achieved when there is concordant imaging with sestamibi and ultrasound scanning in MIP.
- When ioPTH estimation is employed, localization either with sestamibi or USS alone may be fine for MIP.

Ultrasound Scanning

- USS of the parathyroid is low cost, relatively easy to perform, has no radiation exposure, and identifies the parathyroid tumor in about 50–65 % of patients.
- It can be used immediately pre-op in the anesthetic room or on the theatre table. Identifying the location of the parathyroid in relation to the thyroid lobe can aid in sighting the operative incision. It is a very useful tool for the dedicated parathyroid surgeon to learn to use (Figs. 32.1, 32.2, 32.3, 32.4a, b, 32.5, and 32.6a–c).
- USS scanning is more likely to be negative where superior tumors have prolapsed behind the inferior thyroid artery to drop behind the esophagus and when the tumor is in the thymus.

Sestamibi

- Scanning with 99-Tc-sestamibi is the most reliable way to identify parathyroid tumors preoperatively.
- In experienced centers, approximately 60–70 % of patients have a positive scan. SPECT increases the sensitivity of the scan by about 10 % and may be combined with CT scanning.
- When USS and sestamibi scans are concordant in identifying a single adenoma, there is about a 98 % likelihood that removing the tumor will result in cure for the patient.

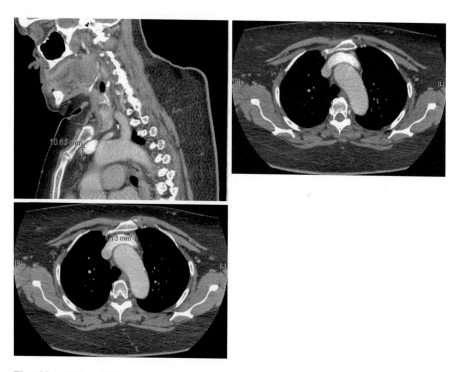

Figs. 32.1, 32.2, and 32.3 Small mediastinal parathyroid adenoma on a contrast-enhanced CT

- Sestamibi scans are more likely to be negative in small tumors (<500 mg), in multigland disease, and in parathyroid hyperplasia (renal disease, MEN).

As the expected cure rate of >95 % is anticipated even in non-localized patients for first-time parathyroid surgery, the significant additional cost incurred in performing other imaging (CT, MRI) as a matter of routine preoperatively is prohibitive, adds little value, and is not recommended.

Localization for Reoperative Surgery

When reoperative surgery is planned for persistent or recurrent hyperparathyroidism, localization studies should be considered mandatory in all patients. The algorithm used by the author is:

- USS
- SPECT/CT
- MRI

    - CT angiography if all above are negative
    - Selective venous catheterization studies if all above negative

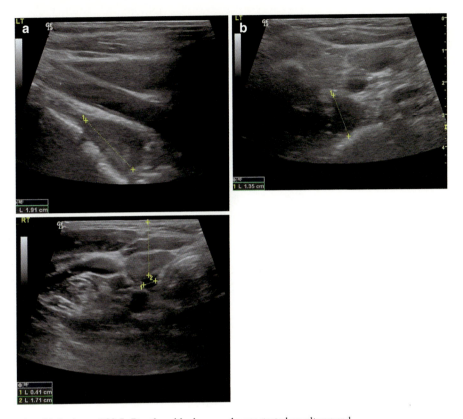

Figs. 32.4a, b, and 32.5 Parathyroid adenoma demonstrated on ultrasound

SPECT/CT

Functional scanning with single photon emission computed tomography (SPECT) when combined with anatomical information in the form of a hybrid SPECT/CT scanner is a recent development. SPECT increases sensitivity over sestamibi scanning alone by about 10 %. Scanners are expensive. When positive, the functional information gained is extremely useful in confirming the suspected lesion seen on CT as a parathyroid (it is often difficult to distinguish parathyroid tissue and lymph nodes on CT).

MRI

In the very difficult situation where sestamibi, CT, and USS scans are all negative, MRI will often identify the missing parathyroid tumor. The author has found MRI to be the most useful tool in identifying parathyroid tumors in patients needing

Fig. 32.6 (**a**, **b**) T1-weighted MRIs of a small parathyroid adenoma. (**c**) The same parathyroid adenoma as (**a**) on fatsat T2-weighted imaging

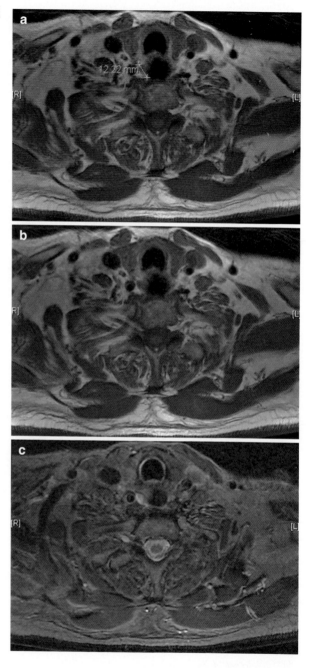

reoperative surgery. An expert radiologist with an interest in endocrine radiology is key. There is the added benefit of no radiation, but some patients are unable to tolerate the claustrophobia of MRI.

CT Angiography

If USS, SPECT/CT, and MRI have failed to locate the missing parathyroid tumor, CT angiography is occasionally useful. Parathyroid tissue has an extremely high vascularity, and it may be possible to demonstrate a "blush" of the tumor in the neck or chest where other imaging modalities have failed. When positive, the information gained from an anatomical perspective for planned operation is extremely useful.

Selective Venous Catheterization (SVC)

When all the above imaging techniques have been tried, consider SVC. This involves placing a femoral catheter, passing the line into the major vessels in the neck and chest, and taking samples for PTH analysis. In the author's experience, once you get to SVC to try and locate a parathyroid tumor, you are clutching at straws. It may be helpful to determine whether levels are high in the neck or chest, but false positives are common and mapping will vary considerably in the same patient when the test is tried at different time intervals.

If all pre-op imaging is completely negative and an experienced parathyroid surgeon has already spent several hours exploring a patient's neck, you are facing perhaps the most difficult of all endocrine operations. In this situation, if the clinical circumstances allow, the author prefers to wait and repeat the tests again at a suitable interval. Occasionally, you get lucky and find that a sestamibi scan previously negative becomes positive or the tumor is seen on MRI or CT angiogram.

Further Reading

Bilezikian JP, Khan AA, Potts JT. Guidelines for the management of asymptomatic primary hyperparathyroidism: summary statement from the third international workshop. J Clin Endocrinol Metab. 2009;94(2):335.

Mihai R, Wass JA, Sadler GP. Asymptomatic hyperparathyroidism–need for multicentre studies. Clin Endocrinol. 2008a;68(2):155–64.

Mihai R, Wass JA, Sadler GP. Pasieka's parathyroid symptoms scores correlate with SF-36 scores in patients undergoing surgery for primary hyperparathyroidism. World J Surg. 2008b;32(5):807–14.

Chapter 33
Surgery for Primary Hyperparathyroidism

R. James England and Hisham Mehanna

Introduction

Primary hyperparathyroidism (PHPT) is the third most common endocrine disorder affecting 0.3 % of the population and up to 1–3 % of postmenopausal women (Jessica et al. 2011).

PHPT is diagnosed by a raised serum (corrected) calcium associated with an inappropriately unsuppressed PTH level. It arises from oversecretion of PTH due to parathyroid gland(s) overactivity.

Primary HPT may be treated conservatively or surgically. Only approximately one-tenth of diagnosed patients end up undergoing parathyroidectomy.

Inherited forms of HPT: Germline mutations leading to loss of heterozygosity in tumor suppressor genes in multiple endocrine neoplasia (MEN)1 and CDC73, combined with a second mutation in somatic cells, can lead to parathyroid tumor development (Jessica et al. 2011).

R.J. England, MBChB, FRCS (ORL-HNS) (✉)
Department of ENT/Head and Neck Surgery,
Hull and East Yorkshire Hospitals NHS Trust,
Castle Hill Hospital, Castle Street, Cottingham,
East Riding of Yorkshire HU16 5JQ, UK
e-mail: rjaeathome@aol.com

H. Mehanna, PhD, BMedSc (hons), MBChB (hons), FRCS, FRCS (ORL-HNS),
Department of Head and Neck Surgery,
School of Cancer Sciences, Institute of Head and Neck Studies and Education,
University of Birmingham, Birmingham, UK

J.C. Watkinson, D.M. Scott-Coombes (eds.), *Tips and Tricks in Endocrine Surgery*,
DOI 10.1007/978-1-4471-2146-6_33, © Springer-Verlag London 2014

Presentation (See Also Chap. 31)

The pattern of presentation has altered radically due to the introduction of the serum autoanalyzer. Most PHPT is now discovered incidentally in primary care in minimally symptomatic patients. Traditionally, the presentation of hyperparathyroidism was labelled as "bones, stones, abdominal groans, and psychic moans." These include bone pain, abdominal pain and cramps, renal stones, and depressed or altered mood.

In the preoperative work-up for all HPT patients, it is important to exclude medically treatable causes of multigland disease by assessing drug history (particularly lithium therapy) and checking for hypovitaminosis D. In addition, a family history of HPT should always be sought, as HPT due to multigland disease is far more likely to be an inherited condition.

Investigations

Investigations aim to confirm a biochemical diagnosis of PHPT and, in minimally symptomatic disease, to identify evidence of end organ damage so that surgery can be recommended.

All patients presenting with a likely diagnosis of PHPT require a serum calcium and intact PTH assay. In addition a serum vitamin D assay is required, and occasionally vitamin D levels must be replete before the diagnosis can be accurately made.

Although hypercalciuria is no longer an indication to advise parathyroidectomy, a 24 h urine collection for calcium and creatinine should still be obtained to exclude the diagnosis of familial hypercalcemic hypocalciuria (see Chap. 31).

Bone density assessment should be considered, particularly in conservatively managed patients to provide a baseline for regular monitoring. A renal ultrasound is performed to determine the presence of renal stones or nephrocalcinosis.

If the need for surgery is established, parathyroid imaging is normally performed (see Chap. 32).

Management

This should always be undertaken in a multidisciplinary setting, in close collaboration with an endocrinologist, preferably specializing in bone metabolism, and ideally with a radiologist specializing in head and neck imaging.

Conservative

Minimally symptomatic patients with no evidence of end organ damage can undergo conservative management with serial observation of calcium, vitamin D, bone density, and renal function. This is especially applicable to patients over the age of 65.

However, up to a third of these patients, when monitored in the long term, develop overt symptoms of hyperparathyroidism.

In patients who are unfit for surgery, long-term follow-up with organ protection and symptom minimization is the aim. This is achieved by the appropriate use of calcimimetics and bisphosphonates. This therapy can prove costly and the side effect profiles of the drugs used may be high.

Surgical Management

It has been shown that successful parathyroidectomy results in restoring bone density suggesting that fracture risk reduces.

Indications for Surgery

In surgically suitable patients, parathyroid surgery is recommended in symptomatic hyperparathyroidism and is advised in asymptomatic compliant patients using guidelines most recently updated in 2008 (Bilezikian et al. 2009) (see Chaps. 31 and 32).

Surgery is also recommended for patients where monitoring is either not desired or possible.

Surgery for a localized single parathyroid adenoma is now usually performed via minimally invasive parathyroidectomy (MIP) (see Chap. 34).

Absolute Indications for Open or Four-Gland Exploration:

1. Previously failed parathyroid exploration
2. Previous surgery to the thyroid on that side of the neck

Relative Indications:

1. Failure to localize overactive parathyroid tissue preoperatively (this is still possible via MIP if performed by an experienced surgeon)
2. A large adenoma that cannot be removed through a 1.5 cm incision

Tips for Surgery

The maintenance of a bloodless field is essential as identification of parathyroid glands, particularly if suppressed, may depend on subtle color differences. This can be facilitated by head elevation and hypotensive anesthesia.

Some surgeons use an *i.v.* infusion of methylene blue (7.5 mg/kg) in 500 ml saline 1 h before operation to localize the parathyroid intraoperatively.

Start to look for the more consistently located superior gland. 80 % of superior parathyroids are found in a one centimeter radius above the intersection of the inferior thyroid artery with the recurrent laryngeal nerve. Most (70 %) of inferior parathyroids are found around the lower pole of the thyroid lobe in the thyrothymic tract – a condensation of fascia between the thyroid and thymic glands.

As the blood supply to the parathyroids is predominantly from the inferior thyroid artery, tracing this medially will often reveal an elusive gland.

Always consider the plane in which the glands lie. The superior glands lie posterior and deep to the recurrent nerve, but when the thyroid lobe is retracted medially, the relationship is inverted and the gland becomes superficial to the recurrent nerve. The inferior gland lies in a plane superficial to the nerve, as does the thymus which is medial to the nerve at the level of the thoracic inlet.

Aim to mobilize the ipsilateral thyroid lobe up and onto the trachea as much as possible prior to searching for the glands as this enables a thorough search deep to the lobe.

If a gland remains undiscovered on one side, locating the contralateral matching gland is recommended as the glands are symmetrical in 80 % of cases.

If a superior gland remains undiscovered, consider the following:

A retro-esophageal adenoma, particularly on the right side. This is usually evidenced by a fatty fullness above the recurrent nerve in the portion within 1 cm of Berry's ligament. Other ectopic positions to consider include the paraesophageal gutter and the carotid sheath.

The superior pole should be mobilized and examined posteromedially between the cricothyroid muscle and the pole itself.

If an inferior gland remains undiscovered, a transcervical thymectomy should be performed.

If a gland still remains undiscovered:

(a) Consider an intrathyroidal gland, but do not undertake a "blind" hemithyroidectomy.
(b) Consider ligating the inferior thyroid artery laterally as this may devascularize an adenoma and make it more visually evident due to color change.
(c) Stop the operation. If there is obvious lymphadenopathy, perform a biopsy to exclude sarcoidosis.
(d) Go over all of the evidence and consider further localization studies.

Complications and Outcomes

Following successful parathyroidectomy, a minority of patients will develop transient symptoms of hypocalcemia for days to weeks. If unpleasant, calcium tablets in the short term will ameliorate these symptoms.

Following successful parathyroidectomy, intact PTH levels will remain elevated in up to 20 % of cases. This is not a sign of parathyroidectomy failure.

Possible complications include hematoma, vocal cord palsy, and persistent or recurrent HPT (see Chap. 35).

Parathyroid Cancer

Parathyroid cancer is the cause of primary hyperparathyroidism in less than 1 % of cases.

The diagnosis of parathyroid cancer can be difficult to make and is most often made postoperatively during histopathological analysis. The diagnosis should be suspected in a patient with severe hypercalcemia (over 3.5 mmol/l) and an extremely high serum PTH (>10 × the upper limit of the normal range has a positive predictive value of 84 % (Schaapveld et al. 2011)), particularly if a palpable neck mass is evident in the thyroid bed.

Parathyroid cancer is relatively radioresistant and the primary treatment modality is surgical resection. When the diagnosis is suspected, en bloc resection of the parathyroid tumor and the thyroid lobe should be undertaken. Postoperative radiotherapy should be discussed in the MDT meeting.

Multigland Disease

Parathyroid hyperplasia is the cause of primary HPT in approximately 15 % of cases. Double adenoma in 1–2 % of cases.

When a diagnosis of multigland disease is made, always consider MEN1 and less frequently familial HPT, MEN2A, and HPT jaw tumor syndrome.

Inherited Multigland Disease

MEN1

Autosomal dominant due to mutations of the MEN1 gene on chromosome 11, comprising tumors of parathyroid, pancreas, and pituitary (with associated lipomas, adrenocortical and carcinoid tumors). PHPT is the most common manifestation and should be treated first. It tends to present in a younger age group and affects 95 % of patients by the age of 30 years.

Due to genetic programming the condition will inevitably recur and therefore the surgical aim is to undertake a subtotal parathyroidectomy and prepare for recurrence.

In most hands the operation of choice is a subtotal parathyroidectomy leaving a well vascularized remnant marked with either clip or a prolene suture or both – away from the recurrent laryngeal nerve.

MEN2A

Associated with mild PHPT. It is far less significant than the associated medullary thyroid carcinoma and pheochromocytoma, and the surgical treatment is to remove clinically abnormal glands only.

Hyperparathyroidism Jaw Tumor Syndrome (HPT-JT)

Autosomal dominant due to mutation of CDC73 gene, characterized by HPT which can occur in adolescence associated with fibroosseous jaw tumors, renal lesions, and parathyroid cancer in 15 %.

Surgery involves total parathyroidectomy with autotransplantation or unilateral clearance in the presence of single gland disease to facilitate second surgery and minimize the risk of surgical morbidity.

Severe Neonatal HPT

Due to homozygous CAR gene mutation on chromosome 3. It requires total parathyroidectomy with autotransplantation.

Pearls and Pitfalls
Pearls

- Have a prepared planned surgical strategy if the tumor is not readily localized at operation.
- Look at the localization studies yourself – you may see something that the radiologist was hesitant to "call."
- Use of a headlight greatly enhances the operative view.
- When a tumor is localized, start the mobilization laterally – it tends to be avascular.
- Aim to "dissect the patient from the tumor!"
- Audit your outcomes.

Pitfalls

- Targeted surgery risks missing patients with multiple gland disease.
- Normal parathyroid glands may appear larger in the presence of vitamin D deficiency.
- Most "ectopic" glands are in classically described locations.

References

Bilezikian JP, Khan AA, Potts Jr JT, Third International Workshop on the Management of Asymptomatic Primary Hyperthyroidism. Guidelines for the management of asymptomatic primary hyperparathyroidism: summary statement from the third international workshop. J Clin Endocrinol Metabol. 2009;94(2):335–9.

Jessica MK-F, Sandra S, Donald A, Jibran S, Aneal K. Primary hyperparathyroidism: an overview. Int J Endocrinol. 2011;2011:251410.

Schaapveld M, Jorna FH, Aben KK, Haak HR, Plukker JT, Links TP. Incidence and prognosis of parathyroid gland carcinoma: a population-based study in the Netherlands estimating the preoperative diagnosis. Am J Surg. 2011;202(5):509–7.

Chapter 34
Minimally Invasive Parathyroidectomy

Ioannis Christakis and Fausto Palazzo

Abbreviations

BNE	Bilateral neck exploration
FAA	Focused anterior approach
FLA	Focused lateral approach
GA	General anesthesia
IOPTH	Intraoperative PTH
LA	Local anesthesia
MEN	Multiple endocrine neoplasia
MGD	Multiple gland disease
MIP	Minimally invasive parathyroidectomy
MIVAT	Video-assisted parathyroidectomy
NIH	National Institute of Health
PET	Positron emission tomography
pHPT	Primary hyperparathyroidism
PTH	Parathyroid hormone
SCM	Sternocleidomastoid muscle
SPECT	Single-photon emission computed tomography
US	Ultrasound

I. Christakis • F. Palazzo (✉)
Department of Thyroid and Endocrine Surgery,
Imperial College NHS Trust,
Hammersmith Campus, London, UK
e-mail: f.palazzo@imperial.ac.uk

J.C. Watkinson, D.M. Scott-Coombes (eds.), *Tips and Tricks in Endocrine Surgery*,
DOI 10.1007/978-1-4471-2146-6_34, © Springer-Verlag London 2014

Introduction

The operative management of primary hyperparathyroidism has changed significantly since the first parathyroidectomy performed almost a century ago (Delbridge and Palazzo 2007). The standard procedure has evolved over decades into the bilateral neck exploration (BNE) which involves the careful identification of all parathyroid glands. Abnormal glands are removed and the normal glands are left in situ without biopsy.

The BNE has the advantage of:

- Allowing the direct visualization of all parathyroid glands
- Immediate management of all scenarios: double adenomas, hyperplasia, ectopic glands, supernumerary glands, etc.
- Minimal morbidity and no mortality

Since over 85 % of pHPT is caused by a single adenoma, the possibility of focusing on the removal of the single abnormal gland and avoiding extra dissection and manipulation of normal parathyroid glands could prevent the risk of complications including hypoparathyroidism, recurrent laryngeal nerve damage, and bleeding. This is the theoretical platform on which focused parathyroid surgery is based.

Focused parathyroid surgery was for many years hindered by the lack of accurate and reliable preoperative localization methods. Neck ultrasonography and technetium-thallium scanning tried to address that problem but the results were patchy. The key breakthroughs in focused parathyroid surgery were:

- The arrival of Tc-99 m sestamibi scanning in 1989
- Improvements in ultrasound scanning and radiological specialization
- The development of intraoperative quick PTH

  - Assays based on two-site antibody immune-radiometric assay by Nussbaum and the two-site immune-chemiluminometric assay by Brown et al.

The pioneering results obtained with the use of focused unilateral surgery (Sidhu et al. 2003) combined with the use of modern technology resulted in the development of various minimally invasive parathyroidectomy (MIP) techniques:

- Focused lateral mini incision
- Endoscopic
- Radio guided
- Video assisted
- Robotic

Imaging Studies and Preoperative Localization (See Chap. 32)

MIP requires accurate preoperative localization of the offending gland(s). Traditionally, localization has been done with the use of ultrasound and $^{99mTc\text{-}sestamibi}$ scan. Other methods that can be of value are computer tomography (CT), magnetic resonance imaging (MRI), and $^{201}Tl/^{99m}Tc$ sodium pertechnetate scanning. Other methods such as intravenous jugular sampling are reserved for cases where the other methods are non-corcodant or negative.

Minimally Invasive Parathyroidectomy

Contraindications to All MIP Modalities

1. History of neck irradiation and prior neck surgery
2. Concomitant multinodular goiter
3. Diagnosis of multiple endocrine neoplasia
4. Proven autoimmune thyroiditis (relative contraindication)
5. Suspicion of carcinoma
6. Anatomic considerations such as extreme obesity

MIP Modalities

Focused Lateral Approach (FLA)

- The most popular technique worldwide
- Can be done under local anesthesia (LA) or general anesthesia (GA)
- Technique:
  - Positioning of the patient:
    - The same as for any thyroid operation – avoid neck overextension.
  - A 2 cm incision is made over the anterior border of the sternocleidomastoid muscle (SCM) and the lateral border of the strap muscles (Agarwal et al. 2002).
  - After dissecting through the subcutaneous fat and platysma, the investing layer of deep cervical fascia is incised.
  - The strap muscles are retracted to expose the thyroid.
  - After identification of the recurrent laryngeal nerve (for superior glands). the offending adenoma is excised.

Focused Anterior Approach (FAA)

- The FAA shares many common characteristics with the lateral approach, differing only in the actual site of incision and the plane of dissection.
  - 2–3 cm transverse incision in the midline
  - Separation of strap muscles
  - Approaching the parathyroid lesion similarly to the conventional exploration (Udelsman and Donovan 2004)

- This technique gives easy access to the inferior parathyroid glands of both sides, but the superior glands may be difficult to approach, especially if they are located posteriorly.

Radio-Guided Parathyroidectomy

- Uses a radiotracer that when administered, accumulates preferentially in the parathyroid glands.
  - 99mTc-sestamibi is used, given in a dose of 10 mCi intravenous, usually 1–2 h before the operation.
  - The radiotracer is detected by the use of an intraoperative gamma probe which guides the dissection.
  - A one stop method has been employed in which patients are injected with a dose of 20 mCi and have a scintigraphy and an operation on the same day (Norman and Chheda 1997).
- The operation can be done under GA or under LA using local anesthetic (lidocaine, 1 % with epinephrine) and intravenous sedation (propofol).
- Technique:
  - The 2–4 cm incision site is based on the data of the sestamibi scan and the radiotracer emissions on the skin as detected by the probe. The incision allows for extension in cases of inadequate operative space and conversion to BNE.
  - The dissection is then guided by the readings of the probe which consist of the radiotracer counts compared to the background counts.
  - The counts recorded while dissecting "in vivo counts" are expressed as a percentage of the background counts.
  - When this in vivo percentage is more than 150 %, a parathyroid adenoma is very likely.
  - After excision, the removed parathyroid gland radioactivity is measured – "ex vivo count."
  - If there is a difference of 20 % or higher between ex vivo and background counts, the operation is complete and no further need to identify the ipsilateral gland is required (Mariani et al. 2003).

Video-Assisted Parathyroidectomy (MIVAT)

- First described by Miccoli et al. in (1998).
- Carried out under GA or under bilateral superficial cervical block in association with laryngeal mask and sevoflurane administration. The surgical team in addition to the scrub nurse comprises three members – surgeon, cameraman, retractor.

- Technique:
    - A 15-mm transverse incision is made above the sternal notch.
    - After dissection of the cervical midline, retractors are inserted and a 5-mm 30° scope inserted to guide the dissection.
    - The magnification provided by the endoscope allows easier identification of the parathyroid glands and the recurrent laryngeal nerve.

Endoscopic Parathyroidectomy

- Gagner in 1996 first described a full endoscopic technique, but it was criticized for its increased operative time and the occurring surgical emphysema (Gagner 1996).
- The lateral endoscopic technique was described and popularized by Henry in Marseille (1999).
- Technique:
    - A 5- or 10-mm fiber-optic endoscope and two 2.5-mm trocars are used.
    - The procedure is performed with the patient in a supine position under GA. The three trocars are placed on the anterior border of the SCM on the side of the lesion.
    - An initial 12- to 15-mm transversal skin crease incision is made on the anterior border of the SCM similar to the focused lateral approach. After division of the platysma, the investing layer of cervical fascia is incised. Dissection is continued to the prevertebral fascia.
    - Three trocars are inserted: a 10-mm trocar through the incision and two 2.5-mm trocars above and below the main optic trocar.
    - Low-pressure (8 mmHg) insufflation with carbon dioxide (CO_2) begins under endoscopic vision.
    - Blunt dissectors are used to mobilize the thyroid lobe and identify the offending parathyroid adenoma which is then removed following control of the pedicle.
- Alternative endoscopic approaches designed to avoid neck scars such as the axillary approach have failed to gather exponents in the West. This is due to the very long operating times and extensive dissection required for access.

Robotic Parathyroidectomy

- Positioning of the patient: Similar to traditional parathyroidectomy with neck extension, ipsilateral arm flexed at shoulder and internally rotated at elbow joint over the head, in order to provide optimal exposure of the axillary region.

- Technique:

  - A 5–6-cm longitudinal incision is made along the outer border of pectoralis major muscle.
  - Skin flaps superficial to pectoralis fascia are extended towards the clavicle and the sternal notch.
  - Strap muscle separation from thyroid capsule under direct vision and insertion of the robotic arms with a 30-mm camera.
  - A robotic retractor elevates the strap musculature and maintains the working space.
  - The technique of parathyroidectomy itself remains the same (Landry et al. 2011).

- Alternatively:

  - Dissection begins through the sternal and clavicular heads of SCM from a small infraclavicular ipsilateral incision.
  - Three trocars are inserted through small incisions made in the anterior axillary line accommodating a 0° dual channel endoscope and two 5-mm robotic instruments.

- Robotic-assisted thoracoscopic techniques have already been used, with relative success, in the excision of mediastinal parathyroid tumors (Ismail et al. 2010).

It remains to be seen if the advantages of 3D-magnified dissection, no need for CO_2 insufflation and a scarless neck area, can outweigh the increased cost of the procedure and the longer operating times.

Intraoperative PTH (IOPTH)

- Principle: If a diseased parathyroid gland is removed, there is a fall in the levels of the circulating PTH measureable in minutes.
- Blood samples are taken intraoperatively from an intravenous peripheral line.

  - First sample: Baseline, at time of anesthesia
  - Second sample: Prior to the excision of the adenoma
  - Third sample: 5 min after excision
  - Fourth sample: 10 min afterwards
  - Fifth sample (optional): 15 min afterwards

- Different criteria exist in order to interpret the data collected.

Criteria for IOPTH Decline (Barczynski et al. 2009)

Miami: Drop of 50 % or more from the highest of either preoperative baseline or pre-excision level 10 min after removal
Vienna: Drop of 50 % or greater from the pre-incision value within 10 min after resection

Rome: Greater than 50 % from the highest pre-excision level, and/or IOPTH concentration within the reference range at 20 min post-excision, and/or less than or equal to 7.5 ng/L lower than the value at 10 min post-excision

Halle: Drop into low-normal range within 15 min after removal

Since MIP does not involve the routine identification of all glands, IOPTH theoretically prevents failure to cure.

- While IOPTH is highly valuable in difficult situations such as re-operations, the only proven documented advantages of the use of IOPTH are a slight improvement of the cure rates and the possible shortening of operative time (Miura et al. 2002).
- IOPTH seems to be less accurate in cases of:

  1. Multi-gland disease (MGD), thus giving false positive results
  2. Anesthetic agents such as propofol are used.
  3. When the patient is under lithium treatment

- The cost-benefit ratio of IOPTH in primary parathyroid surgery is questionable (Agarwal et al. 2001).

Local Versus General Anesthesia

- General anesthesia (GA) for parathyroidectomy is a very safe and routine procedure.

  - With experience of minimal invasive techniques, local anesthesia (LA) has been adopted in increasing numbers of patients.

- If cervical block is used, an injection of 1 % lidocaine is made along the posterior border of the SCM muscle, ipsilateral to the site of the operation. A total volume of 20 ml of 1 % lidocaine is injected at a depth of no greater than 1 cm, in order to block the anterior cervical, the supraclavicular, and the greater auricular nerves.
- LA technique, without cervical block, uses only lidocaine to create a local field block over the incision site. Additional local anesthetic is being injected progressively as the dissection reaches deeper levels.
- Propofol and fentanyl citrate are the most commonly used agents to provide sedation.

Conclusions

- Minimally invasive parathyroidectomy is now the co-gold standard with the bilateral neck exploration when the parathyroid disease is localized. It is safe and can provide results equivalent to open surgery.
- The advantages include a high cure rate, low complication rate, reduced pain, and better cosmetic results. There is also a possible decrease in cost due to shorter hospital stays.

Bibliography

Agarwal G, Barakate MS, Robinson B, Wilkinson M, Barraclough B, Reeve TS, et al. Intraoperative quick parathyroid hormone versus same-day parathyroid hormone testing for minimally invasive parathyroidectomy: a cost-effectiveness study. Surgery. 2001;130:963–70.

Agarwal G, Barraclough BH, Reeve TS, Delbridge LW. Minimally invasive parathyroidectomy using the 'focused' lateral approach. II. Surgical technique. ANZ J Surg. 2002;72:147–51.

Barczynski M, Konturek A, Hubalewska-Dydejczyk A, Cichon S, Nowak W. Evaluation of Halle, Miami, Rome, and Vienna intraoperative iPTH assay criteria in guiding minimally invasive parathyroidectomy. Langenbecks Arch Surg. 2009;394(5):843–9.

Delbridge LW, Palazzo FF. First parathyroid surgeon: Sir John Bland-Sutton and the parathyroids. ANZ J Surg. 2007;77(12):1058–61.

Gagner M. Endoscopic parathyroidectomy. Br J Surg. 1996;83:875.

Henry JF, Defechereux T, Gramatica L, De Boissezon C. Endoscopic parathyroidectomy via a lateral neck incision. Ann Chir. 1999;53:302–6.

Ismail M, Maza S, Swierzy M, Tsilimparis N, Rogalla P, Sandrock D, et al. Resection of ectopic mediastinal parathyroid glands with the da Vinci robotic system. Br J Surg. 2010;97:337–43.

Landry CS, Grubbs EG, Morris GS, Turner NS, Holsinger FC, Lee JE, et al. Robot assisted trans-axillary surgery (RATS) for the removal of thyroid and parathyroid glands. Surgery. 2011;149(4):549–55.

Mariani G, Gulec SA, Rubello D, Boni G, Puccini M, Pelizzo MR, et al. Preoperative localization and radioguided parathyroid surgery. J Nucl Med. 2003;44(9):1443–58.

Miccoli P, Bendinelli C, Conte M, Pinchera A, Marcocci C. Endoscopic parathyroidectomy by a gasless approach. J Laparoendosc Adv Surg Tech A. 1998;8:189–94.

Miura D, Wada N, Arici C, Morita E, Duh QY, Clark OH. Does intraoperative quick parathyroid hormone assay improve the results of parathyroidectomy? World J Surg. 2002;26(8):926–30.

Norman J, Chheda H. Minimally invasive parathyroidectomy facilitated by intraoperative nuclear mapping. Surgery. 1997;122(6):998–1003.

Sidhu S, Neill AK, Russell CF. Long-term outcome of unilateral parathyroid exploration for primary hyperparathyroidism due to presumed solitary adenoma. World J Surg. 2003;27(3):339–42.

Udelsman R, Donovan PI. Open minimally invasive parathyroid surgery. World J Surg. 2004;28(12):1224–6.

Chapter 35
Reoperative Parathyroid Surgery

Thomas W.J. Lennard

Introduction

Firstly establish if this is persistent or recurrent disease:

- Persistent hyperparathyroidism is defined as a failure to correct hypercalcemia after neck exploration and/or removal of a presumed adenoma. This is most commonly due to multiglandular disease or an unsuspected second adenoma.
- Recurrent disease is defined as further evidence of hyperparathyroidism after a previously successful parathyroidectomy greater than 6 months earlier.

These are amongst the most challenging cases for the endocrine surgeon. Therefore it is important to confirm that the patient has symptoms that justify further surgery or evidence of secondary end organ damage from hyperparathyroidism by way of bone disease or renal stones.

Reoperation should only be considered if the patient is symptomatic or there is objective evidence of progressive disease, bone or renal, which justifies the risks and uncertainties of further surgery.

The operating surgeon should consider whether this could be a patient with a predisposition to multiglandular disease such as MEN1 or MEN2. A family history of endocrine syndromes or other components of these syndromes such as pituitary, adrenal, or pancreatic tumors should be sought because recurrent hyperparathyroidism raises the real possibility of an underlying predisposition syndrome.

T.W.J. Lennard, MBBS, FRCS, MD
Department of Surgery, Royal Victoria Infirmary,
Queen Victoria Road, Newcastle Upon Tyne NE1 4PL, UK
e-mail: thomas.lennard@ncl.ac.uk

J.C. Watkinson, D.M. Scott-Coombes (eds.), *Tips and Tricks in Endocrine Surgery*,
DOI 10.1007/978-1-4471-2146-6_35, © Springer-Verlag London 2014

Investigations

Biochemistry

The diagnosis of hyperparathyroidism should be reconfirmed. It will be important to make sure that familial hypercalcemic hypocalciuria has been excluded and that the patient is vitamin D replete. It is essential to repeat biochemical tests and ensure that the calcium is above the normal range and that there is an inappropriately detectable parathyroid hormone level.

All previous investigations including biochemistry, imaging, and most importantly the first and any subsequent operation note should be reviewed making a note of any pathology specimens sent and any results. Using this information, a "road map" of the known and unknown gland positions in the neck should be drawn and a deduction made where the most likely target could be.

Localization (See also Chap. 32)

Re-imaging the neck will then be essential. This will require an ultrasound, a MIBI scan, and an MRI. In addition, selective venous sampling can be of use in this setting. For any abnormalities that are seen on ultrasound, one should consider biopsy under ultrasound control and sending the aspirate for a PTH analysis. This can allow confirmation of any suspect nodules in accessible areas of the neck as being parathyroid tissue.

Reoperations should only be considered if there is concordant localization by at least two indirect modalities or a positive aspirate on one modality.

Preoperative Considerations

The patient should be consented carefully. Redo operations have a higher risk of complications including hemorrhage and vocal cord palsy, and in addition, imaging might be misleading and you may not find the proposed abnormality, leading to failure to cure.

Consider the possibility if extensive previous surgery has been performed [including on occasions and not to be encouraged blind hemithyroidectomy and removal of normal parathyroids] that the only remaining parathyroid tissue in the patient could be the target you intend to remove. Taking care to monitor, therefore, for severe hypoparathyroidism postoperatively will be important.

The patient should have a preoperative vocal cord inspection.

Operative Tips

The operation will be a directed surgery aiming to find only the pre-identified target. If this is in the neck, consider asking your radiologist to place a skin marker over the site of the presumed adenoma or do an on-table ultrasound yourself to guide you for your incision.

Try to approach the gland through virgin territory or tissues. The back door approach, lateral to the strap muscles, is useful if a full formal neck exploration has been previously performed through an anterior cervicotomy. Alternatively, if a focused approach or minimally invasive incision has been used for the previous parathyroid operation, then a new focused approach down to the target would be appropriate.

All tools that can confirm that you have successfully completed the operation should be used including intraoperative PTH measurement and frozen section, and consider having a colleague experienced in endocrine surgery to assist you for this difficult operation. If you do not find the expected adenoma, avoid "blind" hemithyroidectomy or the unselected resection or biopsy of normal parathyroid glands. If unsuccessful, stop the operation before any harm is done, note carefully any findings, and plan to reinvestigate another day.

Pearls and Pitfalls
Pearls

- Know what you are going for.
- Review all previous results before embarking on the operation.
- Consent for possible complications.
- Focus the operation on the target.
- Approach through virgin territory if possible.
- Do everything you can to confirm the success of the operation perioperatively.

Pitfalls

- Avoid operating on the asymptomatic patient or the patient who has no evidence of harm from their further hyperparathyroidism.
- Avoid operating without a clear target to go for.
- Ensure that you have good assistance, plenty of time, and a clear strategy in mind before you start this procedure.
- Failure to take into account the above will make the operation more ... etc.

Further Reading

Fayet P, Heoffel C, Fulla Y, et al. Technetium-99m sestamibi MRI and venous blood sampling in persistent and recurrent hyperparathyroidism. Br J Radiol. 1997;70(833):459–64.

Inabnet WB, Lee JA, Palmer BJA. Parathyroid disease. In: A companion to specialist surgical practice. Endocrine surgery. 5th ed. Saunders: Elsevier; 2014.

Kivlen MH, Bartlett DL, Libutti SK, et al. Reoperation for hyperparathyroidism in MEN. Surgery. 2001;130(6):991–8.

Thompson NW, Eckhauser FE, Harness JK. The anatomy of primary hyperparathyroidism. Surgery. 1982;92(5):814–21.

Weber C, Burke GJ, McGarity WC. Persistent and recurrent sporadic primary hyperparathyroidism: histopathology, complications and results of reoperation. Surgery. 1994;116(6):991–8.

Chapter 36
Renal Hyperparathyroidism

David M. Scott-Coombes

Definitions and Pathophysiology

- On the surface of every parathyroid cell are calcium-sensing receptors (CaSR) (set to 2.20–2.60 mmol/l).
- A fall in serum calcium or a rise in serum phosphate triggers the secretion of parathyroid hormone (PTH).
- PTH has actions on intestines, bone, and kidneys which all result in increased serum calcium until normal physiological concentration has been restored.
- PTH stimulates the second hydroxylation of vitamin D (in the kidney) to produce active vitamin D_3 (calcitriol). Intestinal absorption of calcium can only occur in the presence of both PTH and calcitriol.
- A chronic excess secretion of PTH is termed hyperparathyroidism (HPT).

Secondary hyperparathyroidism (2HPT) results from an appropriate excess secretion of PTH in response to prolonged reduction in serum calcium. The patient has a high PTH with normal calcium. Vitamin D deficiency is the commonest underlying cause, which may be either dietary or secondary to renal failure.

The term *renal hyperparathyroidism* is reserved for those patients with renal failure-induced HPT. The principal mechanisms of renal HPT are:

- Reduced GFR resulting in phosphate retention which binds (and reduces) serum calcium.
- Hyperphosphatemia stimulates PTH secretion.
- A failure to activate calcitriol leading to a reduction in intestinal absorption of calcium.

D.M. Scott-Coombes, MS, FRCS
Department of Endocrine Surgery, University Hospital of Wales,
Heath Park, Cardiff CF14 4XW, UK
e-mail: david.scott-coombes@wales.nhs.uk

J.C. Watkinson, D.M. Scott-Coombes (eds.), *Tips and Tricks in Endocrine Surgery*,
DOI 10.1007/978-1-4471-2146-6_36, © Springer-Verlag London 2014

Most patients are normocalcemic, but some develop hypercalcemia. To avoid confusion, alternative terms are normocalcemic and hypercalcemic renal hyperparathyroidism.

Tertiary hyperparathyroidism (3HPT) is reserved for patients who after a period of dialysis undergo successful renal transplantation, and the previously appropriate excess secretion of PTH (2HPT) becomes inappropriate and results in hypercalcemia – probably due to development of parathyroid adenoma.

Management

The majority of patients can be managed by medical treatment, for which there are several available modalities including:

- Low-phosphate diet
- Phosphate binders
- Active vitamin D sterols
- Calcimimetics

whereby the goal is to maintain optimal PTH level while maintaining controlled serum phosphate and calcium with normal bone turnover rates. Calcimimetics bind to the CaSR and reduce PTH secretion.

Surgery is indicated in patients with advanced renal HPT refractory to medical treatment. However, precise definitions are not simple to describe, but include:

- Inability to maintain calcium or phosphate within a target range
- Inability to decrease a high level of PTH (>50 pmol/l) by more than 50 % after two months of medical therapy
- The presence of symptoms (bone and joint pain, pruritis, muscle weakness, psychiatric irritability)
- Failed treatment by calcimimetics (poor compliance, side effects, failure of PTH to fall, tachyphyllaxis or escape)
- Calciphylaxis: a poorly understood and very morbid syndrome of vascular calcification and skin necrosis (Fig. 36.1)

Better medical control and the introduction of calcimimetics have significantly reduced the need for parathyroidectomy, but it is estimated that up to 10 % of patients may require surgery after 10–15 years of renal replacement therapy. The efficacy of parathyroidectomy in calciphylaxis is uncertain, but may have a role in patients with severe hypercalcemia that do not respond to calcimimetics.

Following successful renal transplantation, most patients become normocalcemic, but it may take several months, and fewer than 5 % of patients will require parathyroidectomy to treat hypercalcemia.

Fig. 36.1 Calciphylaxis in the lower limb

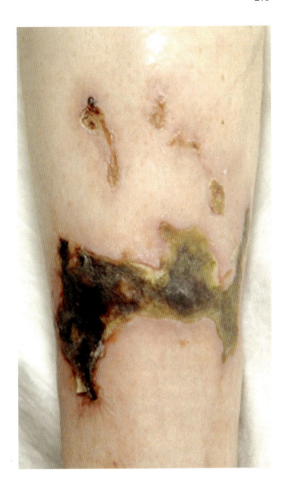

Surgical Options

There is no consensus regarding the optimal surgical procedure for these patients. The literature is hampered by few publications with small numbers of patients, a dearth of randomized studies, and huge variability in the way that the results are presented. There are three available procedures:

- Subtotal parathyroidectomy (sPTX) – excising 3.5 parathyroid glands.
- Total parathyroidectomy with autotransplantation (tPTX + AT) – all four parathyroid glands are excised and a small remnant of minced parathyroid tissue is autotransplanted into the forearm or neck muscle.
- Total parathyroidectomy alone (tPTX) (without autotransplantation) – all four parathyroid glands are excised.

There is no evidence to suggest that any one approach is superior. Recurrence rates for sPTX and tPTX + AT are similar. The latter has the theoretical advantage that redo surgery in the neck could be avoided if the autograft is sited in the forearm. The lowest recurrence rates are seen in tPTX. Even when all parathyroid glands are removed, PTH levels remain detectable, and the theoretical concerns about a dynamic bone disease appear unfounded.

Other factors that influence the operative approach include:

- The likelihood that the patient will receive a kidney transplant
- Patient age and expected survival
- Surgeon's preference

Up to one-third of patients with renal HPT will have supernumerary glands, of which most are in the thymus. Routine thymectomy has been shown to reduce the rate of recurrent HPT.

Surgical Tips

Preoperative

- Close liaison with nephrologists.
- Control hypertension/cardiovascular disease.
- No requirement for radiological parathyroid localization studies for primary surgery.
- Preload with vitamin D 1 week prior to surgery to minimize postoperative hypocalcemia.
- Dialyze close to surgery.

Operation

- Cervicotomy.
- Identify the junction of the recurrent laryngeal nerve and inferior thyroid artery (Fig. 36.2).
- Identify superior glands and excise.
- Identify inferior glands in thyrothymic ligament and excise.
- Perform cervical thymectomy.
- Consider central venous line (for post-op *i.v.* calcium) and a wound drain.
- Close wound.

Postoperative

- Monitor serum calcium closely and replace as necessary.
- May need to increase dose or start vitamin D analogues.

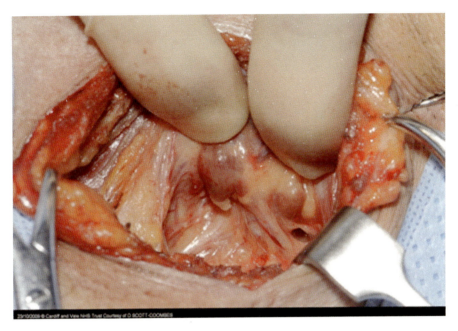

Fig. 36.2 An operative view of the left side of the neck, patient's feet to the left, and head to the right. *ITA* inferior thyroid artery, *RLN* recurrent laryngeal nerve, *IP* inferior parathyroid, *SP* superior parathyroid

- If placed, remove drain on first postoperative day.
- Avoid high-dose heparin with perioperative hemodialysis due to risk of hemorrhage.

Pearls and Pitfalls
- As an aid to localization, remember the symmetry of parathyroid gland pairs.
- To find the thymus, dissect very close to the undersurface of the sternothyroid strap muscle in an inferior (caudal) direction and look for the characteristic whiter opalescent thymic capsule. Then using serial hemostats slowly avulse the thymus from the mediastinum (Fig. 36.3).
- Pay close attention to hemostasis (impaired platelet function in renal failure) and position the patient in Trendelenburg tilt prior to closure.
- DO NOT rupture the capsule as this will place the patient at risk of parathyromatosis – a longer incision may be necessary.

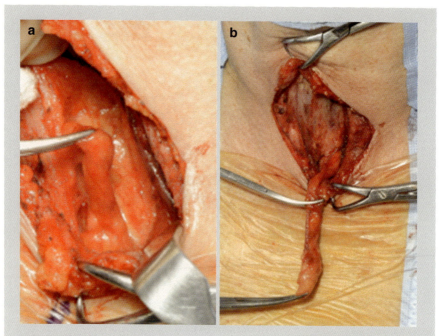

Fig. 36.3 (**a**) Placement of hemostats on thymic horn and slow avulsion. (**b**) Resulting in comprehensive thymectomy

Background Reading

Rothmund M, Wagner PK, Schark C. Subtotal parathyroidectomy versus total parathyroidectomy and autotransplantation in secondary hyperparathyroidism: a randomized trial. World J Surg. 1991;15:745–50.
Saunders RN, Karoo R, Metcalfe MS, Nicholson ML. Four gland parathyroidectomy without reimplantation in patients with chronic renal failure. Postgrad Med J. 2005;81:255–8.
Tominaga Y, Matsuoka S, Uno N. Surgical and medical treatment of secondary hyperparathyroidism in patients on continuous dialysis. World J Surg. 2009;33:2335–42.

Part V
Pituitary

Chapter 37
Presentation and Biochemical Assessment of Pituitary Disease

John Ayuk and Penelope M. Clark

Presentation

Pituitary tumors may present in a number of ways:

(a) Mass effect of the lesion
(b) Pituitary hormone excess
(c) Incidental finding following imaging for an unrelated cause (incidentaloma)

Mass Effect of the Lesion

Usually caused by pituitary macroadenomas (tumors >1 cm in diameter)

J. Ayuk, MD, MRCP
Department of Endocrinology, Queen Elizabeth Hospital
Birmingham, Birmingham, West Midlands B15 2WB, UK

University of Birmingham and Queen Elizabeth Hospital
Birmingham, University Hospital Birmingham NHS Foundation Trust,
Mindelsohn Way, Birmingham B15 2WB, UK
e-mail: john.ayuk@uhb.nhs.uk

P.M. Clark, MSc, PhD, FRCPath (✉)
Regional Endocrine Laboratory, Clinical Laboratory Services,
Queen Elizabeth Hospital Birmingham, Birmingham,
West Midlands B15 2WB, UK

University of Birmingham and Queen Elizabeth Hospital
Birmingham, University Hospital Birmingham NHS Foundation Trust,
Mindelsohn Way, Birmingham B15 2WB, UK
e-mail: p.m.clark@bham.ac.uk

J.C. Watkinson, D.M. Scott-Coombes (eds.), *Tips and Tricks in Endocrine Surgery*,
DOI 10.1007/978-1-4471-2146-6_37, © Springer-Verlag London 2014

Visual Loss

- Bitemporal hemianopia due to compression of the optic chiasm
  Loss of visual acuity due to optic nerve compression
- Changes in color perception
- Diplopia and/or ptosis due to cranial nerve compression

Hypopituitarism

Thyroid Stimulating Hormone (TSH) Deficiency

- Cold intolerance
- Fatigue
- Weight gain
- Constipation
- Pale, dry skin
- Myalgia

Gonadotrophin Deficiency

- Loss of libido
- Infertility
- Loss of body hair
- Amenorrhea, hot flushes, and vaginal dryness in women
- Erectile dysfunction in men

Adrenocorticotrophic Hormone (ACTH) Deficiency

- Fatigue
- Weight loss
- Lethargy
- Hypotension
- Nausea

Growth Hormone (GH) Deficiency

- Growth retardation and short stature in children
- Lethargy and weight gain in adults

Antidiuretic Hormone (ADH) Deficiency

- Diabetes insipidus with polyuria and polydipsia

Pituitary Stalk Compression

- Mild hyperprolactinemia (see symptoms below)

Headache

Pituitary Apoplexy

- Acute pituitary tumor hemorrhage or infarction
- Occurs when tumor outgrows its blood supply
- Sudden onset of symptoms:
  - Headache
  - Visual impairment
  - Altered mental status
- Results in pituitary hormone deficiency

Pituitary Hormone Excess

Hyperprolactinemia

- Oligomenorrhea/amenorrhea in women
- Galactorrhea in women
- Gynecomastia
- Reduced fertility
- Loss of libido
- Erectile dysfunction in men
- Loss of body hair in men

GH Excess (Acromegaly)

- Coarse facial features
- Prognathism and malocclusion
- Enlarged hands and feet
- Headache
- Excess sweating
- Carpal tunnel syndrome
- Snoring and obstructive sleep apnea
- Hypertension
- Glucose intolerance
- Hypertrophic cardiomyopathy
- Osteoarthritis and arthralgia
- Accelerated linear growth (gigantism) if prepubertal

ACTH Excess (Cushing's Disease)

- Centripetal fat distribution, including fat pad over upper part of back
- Exaggerated facial roundness
- Proximal myopathy
- Hypertension
- Easy bruising
- Purple abdominal striae
- Hirsutism
- Osteopenia
- Glucose intolerance
- Neuropsychiatric symptoms

TSH Excess (TSH-Secreting Tumor) – Very Rare

- Weight loss
- Tachycardia and palpitations
- Heat intolerance and excessive sweating
- Hand tremor
- Irritability
- Increased bowel frequency

Gonadotrophin-Secreting Tumor

- Secrete FSH and LH with reduced biological activity
- Most patients present with gonadotrophin deficiency
- Rarely, elevated serum testosterone and testicular enlargement in men
- Rarely, ovarian hyperstimulation and endometrial hyperplasia in women

Pituitary Incidentalomas

Incidental finding following imaging for an unrelated cause
   Two key questions:

- Is the tumor hormonally active?
- Is the tumor causing a mass effect?

Biochemical Assessment

Should precede imaging to avoid the pitfalls of investigation of a pituitary incidentaloma.

Generally, investigation will be performed in conjunction with an endocrinologist with experience of these tests.

Urgent biochemical investigations may be required on presentation. For endocrine tests the appropriate sample should be collected for analysis without delaying treatment. If a result is required for an immediate decision regarding treatment, arrangements should be made with the laboratory.

The aims of biochemical assessment are:

- To determine whether the tumor is functional, i.e., synthesizing and secreting pituitary hormones in an unregulated fashion or whether it is nonfunctional and inappropriate concentrations of circulating hormone are due to pressure effects on the pituitary stalk.
- The outcome of the above investigations should determine whether medical or surgical treatment is appropriate.
- To determine whether the patient is "safe for surgery."
- To determine baseline endocrine function for the long-term management of the patient post surgery.

Basic Investigations

Serum cortisol (Short Synacthen Test), "thyroid function" which for pituitary disease must include both (free) T4 and TSH, and prolactin

Hypothalamic-pituitary-gonadal function – LH/FSH +/– testosterone/estradiol dependant on presentation

Posterior pituitary function; matched serum/urine osmolality and sodium, renal function tests

Dynamic Function Tests

Short Synacthen® Test

Collect basal bloods for serum cortisol and plasma ACTH, administer 250 ug Synacthen im or iv and collect second blood sample for cortisol 30 min later.

Pitfall
ACTH is required for the normal function of the adrenal. Thus, in longstanding pituitary disease, there will be a subnormal adrenal cortisol response. In acute disease or post pituitary surgery, a normal response may be obtained for at least 6 weeks post-insult.

The following tests are generally performed under endocrine supervision.

Oral Glucose Tolerance Test with GH

Consult endocrinologist. Serum insulin-like growth factor-1 (IGF-1) on basal sample. Used for the biochemical diagnosis of acromegaly.

Overnight Dexamethasone Test, Low-/High-Dose Dexamethasone Test, Corticotrophin Releasing Hormone (CRH) Test

Consult endocrinologist. Used for the investigation of Cushing's syndrome.

Water Deprivation Test

Consult endocrinologist. For the investigation of polyuria/polydipsia, namely, posterior pituitary function.

Prolactin

Circulating concentrations are elevated due to stress, many psychotropic drugs, hypothyroidism, and in pregnancy.

If drugs known to cause hyperprolactinemia cannot be withdrawn, imaging is necessary.

A form of prolactin bound to immunoglobulins known as "macroprolactin" can be measured by some prolactin assays giving rise a false elevation. All laboratories should offer a screening test for macroprolactin (usually polyethylene glycol (PEG) precipitation) to exclude it as a cause of a raised prolactin.

The term "macroprolactin" (immunoglobulin-bound prolactin) should not be confused with a "macroprolactinoma" (a large tumor which secretes prolactin).

"Free Hormones"

Changes in the concentrations of proteins that bind hormones are found in pregnancy, oral contraceptive use and complicate the interpretation of some tests.

Affected tests include total thyroxine (thyroxine-binding globulin and albumin), testosterone/estradiol (sex hormone-binding globulin, SHBG), and cortisol (cortisol-binding globulin).

Free thyroxine and SHBG are measured to overcome these effects. Interpretation of cortisol results will need to take these affects into account.

Pearls and Pitfalls
Pearl

- Contact your endocrinologist for advice
- Contact your laboratory particularly for urgent endocrine investigations
- Concentrations of hormones in blood may be given in different units, e.g., GH in ug/L and mIU/L. Remember to check the units of reporting

Pitfall

- Some pituitary tumors secrete more than one hormone; check for all
- Beware of mass effect caused by "non-endocrine" pituitary lesions, e.g., metastases, aneurysms, granulomatous disease
- "Macroprolactin" (immunoglobulin-bound prolactin) should not be confused with "macroprolactinoma"
- Many hormones show a diurnal rhythm
- Many drugs can effect hormone concentrations – exclude these as a cause

Further Reading

Clark PMS, Gordon K. Challenges for the endocrine laboratory in critical illness. Best Pract Res Clin Endocrinol Metab (Cooper MS, Venkatesh B, editors). 2011;25:847–59.

Levy A. Pituitary disease: presentation, diagnosis, and management. J Neurol Neurosurg Psychiatry. 2004;75 Suppl 3:iii47–52.

Molitch ME. Medication-induced hyperprolactinemia. Mayo Clin Proc. 2010;80(8):1050–7.

Wass JAH, Stewart PM, editors. Oxford textbook of endocrinology and diabetes. 2nd ed. Oxford: Oxford University Press; 2011.

Chapter 38
Localization and Imaging of Pituitary Tumors

Lisha McClelland, Shahzada K. Ahmed, and Swarupsinh V. Chavda

Pituitary Imaging

The pituitary gland is best imaged with magnetic resonance imaging (MRI) that will delineate the normal gland and identify any areas of abnormality within the gland. Computed tomography (CT) scans can give additional information about the bony anatomy; however, it requires exposure to radiation and is generally reserved for patients not suitable for MRI, i.e., pacemaker. CT is also utilized for navigation planning in endoscopic sinus surgery.

L. McClelland
Department of Otolaryngology,
Queen Elizabeth Hospital Birmingham,
University Hospital Birmingham NHS Foundation Trust,
Mindelsohn Way, Birmingham B15 2WB, UK

S.K. Ahmed (✉)
Department of Ear, Nose and Throat Surgery,
Queen Elizabeth Hospital Birmingham,
University Hospital Birmingham NHS Foundation Trust,
Mindelsohn Way, Birmingham B15 2WB, UK
e-mail: shahz.ahmed@nhs.net

S.V. Chavda
Department of Neuroradiology,
Queen Elizabeth Hospital Birmingham,
University Hospital Birmingham NHS Foundation Trust,
Mindelsohn Way, Birmingham B15 2WB, UK
e-mail: chavda@uhb.nhs.uk

J.C. Watkinson, D.M. Scott-Coombes (eds.), *Tips and Tricks in Endocrine Surgery*,
DOI 10.1007/978-1-4471-2146-6_38, © Springer-Verlag London 2014

Fig. 38.1 Axial CT scan showing empty sella. CT scan (axial image). Note expanded sella occupied by hypodense CSF, with infundibulum in center

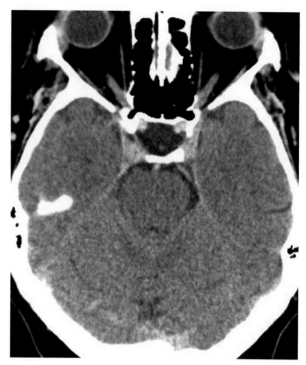

MRI Scan

Pros	Cons
No radiation	Claustrophobia
Multiplanar	Non-MRI-compatible metal
Excellent soft tissue details	Cost
Better resolution	
Tissue differentiation	

MRI Protocol

- T1 sagittal
- Dual-echo axial
- Pre- and post-contrast high-resolution T1 sagittal and coronal to pituitary gland (1 mm or less)
- T2 WI coronal to pituitary gland
- Diffusion-weighted scan – optional
- MR angiogram – optional

CT Scanning

Pros	Cons
Availability	Radiation exposure (reduced with cone beam CT scanners)
Fast	Soft tissue detail inferior to MRI
Relatively inexpensive	
Good bone detail	
Acute bleed/proteinaceous material	
Surgical planning – navigation	

CT scans can provide additional information about the bony margins of the fossa. It may be useful in identifying bone asymmetry, expansion, or erosion if present. Calcification is also easier to identify on CT (Fig. 38.1).

The Pituitary Gland on Imaging

MRI is excellent at delineating the pituitary gland size, shape, and intensity (Fig. 38.2a–d). The anterior gland is isointense with the brain while the posterior gland is hyperintense (bright) on T1. The normal gland should enhance after contrast as there is no blood–brain barrier. Approximately 10 % of glands are asymmetrical and small cysts may be present within a normal gland.

In the surrounding area the clivus is hyperintense on T1 and cortical bone is hypointense (black). The sphenoid sinus is seen as a signal void on all weightings (black). The internal carotid artery is seen as a signal void within the cavernous sinus. The course of the optic nerves to the optic chiasm and optic tracts can be easily identified on MRI.

Microadenoma <1 cm, usually located in pars distalis (Fig. 38.3)
Macroadenoma >1 cm (Fig. 38.4a, b)

- On T1 an adenoma is iso- or hypointense.
- On post-contrast T1 (T1 gadolinium adenoma is hypointense than normal gland and on delayed scan may be iso- or hyperintense).
- Isointense or hypointense on T2 unless cystic.
- Tumor consistency: in general a homogeneous tumor is soft and heterogeneous and more fibrous.
- Tumor above the diaphragm ("cottage loaf," "snow man," or "figure of eight").
- Cavernous sinus invasion.
- Optic nerve compression.
- Bony erosion of the posterior wall of the sphenoid, pituitary fossa, or clivus.

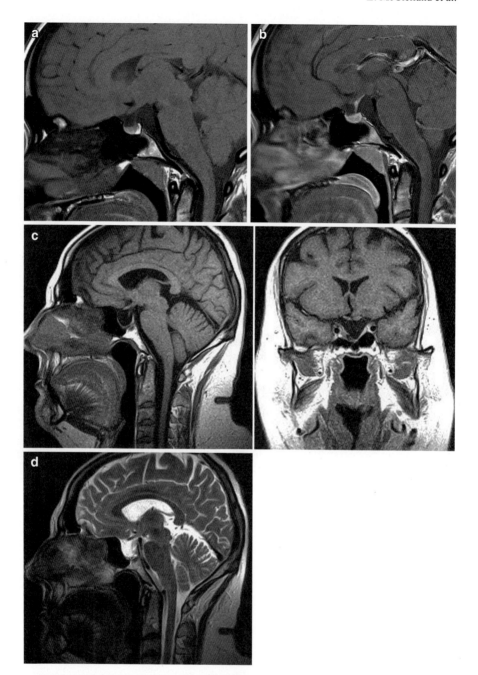

Fig. 38.2 (**a**) Sagittal T1. Normal high signal from the posterior pituitary gland. (**b**) Sagittal post-contrast T1. Normal enhancement of the infundibulum and gland. (**c**) MRI scan. T1 sagittal and coronal scans. Expanded sella occupied by hypointense CSF. (**d**) MRI scan T2 sagittal. Hyperintense CSF occupying sella

Fig. 38.3 Microadenoma (less than 1 cm). Note small (<1 cm) hypointense microadenoma in the left half of the pituitary gland on this post-contrast T1. The pituitary infundibulum is displaced to the right

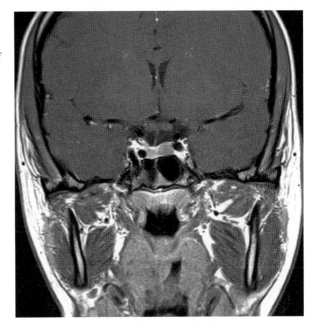

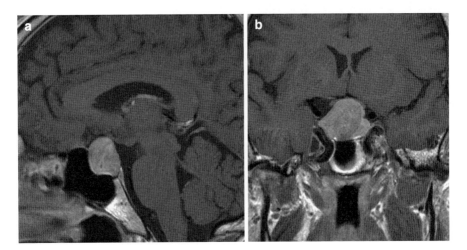

Fig. 38.4 (**a**) Macroadenoma (greater than 1 cm). Pituitary macroadenoma occupying an enlarged sella with suprasella extension. The origin of the tumor is seen to start within the gland. The sphenoid sinus is clear. Tumor shows uniform enhancement on post-contrast sagittal T1. (**b**) Macroadenoma (greater than 1 cm). Coronal post-contrast T1. Note distortion of the optic chiasm and early lateral extension into cavernous sinuses

Craniopharyngioma

Suprasella with small intrasellar component
Solid/cystic component. Calcification common (Fig. 38.5a, b)

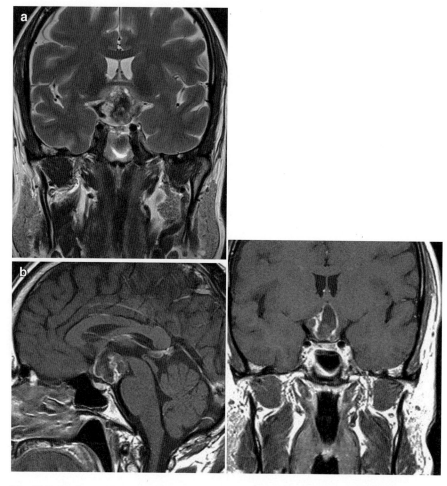

Fig. 38.5 (**a**) Coronal T2. Note the suprasella solid/cystic mass lesion. Signal void due to calcification often seen on imaging. (**b**) Post-contrast T1. Enhancement of the solid component. Note the suprasella position and a normal pituitary gland separate from the tumor

Chapter 39
Diagnostic Work-Up and Nonsurgical Management of Pituitary Disease

Thomas J. Beech and Wiebke Arlt

When to Test

Pituitary lesions are rare with an approximate incidence of 2 per 100,000, although autopsy studies have identified pituitary lesions in 11 % of cases. There are three main groups of patients that require diagnostic assessment for characterization or detection of pituitary disease:

1. Pituitary incidentalomas (by far the most common; patients who undergo cranial imaging for reasons unrelated to pituitary pathology, most commonly headaches, and the imaging coincidentally detects a pituitary nodule)
2. Symptomatic patients (either pituitary mass effect with compromised vision or biochemical effect with clinical signs and symptoms of hormone excess)
3. In certain rare conditions that predispose to pituitary lesions, multiple endocrine neoplasia type 1 (MEN-1) syndrome or Carney complex

T.J. Beech, MBChB, MSc, DOHNS, FRCS (✉)
ENT Department, University Hospital Birmingham,
Birmingham, West Midlands B15 2TH, UK
e-mail: tbeech@nhs.net

W. Arlt, MD, DSc, FRCP, FMedSci
Department of Endocrinology, Centre for Endocrinology,
Diabetes and Metabolism (CEDAM),
School of Clinical and Experimental Medicine,
University of Birmingham, Birmingham,
West Midlands B15 2TT, UK
e-mail: w.arlt@bham.ac.uk

J.C. Watkinson, D.M. Scott-Coombes (eds.), *Tips and Tricks in Endocrine Surgery*,
DOI 10.1007/978-1-4471-2146-6_39, © Springer-Verlag London 2014

What Tests

Biochemical Testing

- For all pituitary lesions (including incidentalomas), blood tests should be performed to assess for hyper- and hyposecretion (see section presentation and biochemical assessment of pituitary disease for specific tests).

Ophthalmology Assessment

- If an MRI scan suggests the pituitary mass is close to the optic nerve or chasm, then formal visual fields should be tested by an ophthalmologist.

Imaging

- MRI in all cases.
- Any pituitary incidentalomas detected on CT should also have an MRI.

Inferior Petrosal Sinus Sampling (IPSS)

- Only used in ACTH-dependent Cushing's syndrome to differentiate between Cushing's disease due to an ACTH secreting pituitary microadenoma and ectopic ACTH secretion after ACTH-dependent Cushing's has been biochemically confirmed.
- Performed by interventional radiologist.

Histopathological Examination of Pituitary Lesion

- Essential in cases where there is a potential for malignancy (but all specimens taken during operative management of a pituitary lesion are sent for histological confirmation).
- Immunostaining can give confirmation or additional information in the case of functional tumors (e.g., for ACTH, TSH).
- A pituitary biopsy should only be undertaken if malignancy of non-pituitary origin is suspected and biochemistry has excluded pituitary hormone excess.

Interpretation

Biochemical Testing

- See presentation and biochemical assessment of pituitary disease section.

Imaging

- See localization and imaging of pituitary tumors section.

Inferior Petrosal Sinus Sampling (IPSS)

- 97 % effective at identifying Cushing's disease.
- Comparison of peripheral and central ACTH levels before and 2 and 5 min after intravenous administration of corticotrophin-releasing hormone (CRH) 100 µg.
- If central ACTH levels are higher than peripheral in a ratio of >2 (pre-CRH administration) or >3 (post-CRH administration), this is indicative of Cushing's disease, i.e., pituitary source of ACTH excess.

Follow-Up of Incidentalomas (According to The Endocrine Society)

Patients that do not require surgery (no optic nerve/chiasm compression, no neurology, no apoplexy, or no hypersecretion of non-prolactin nature) should receive medical follow-up with:

- MRI at 6 months for macroadenoma or 12 months for microadenoma
- Follow-up scans yearly (if no growth) thereafter for 3 years, then less frequently
- Visual fields only if signs of optic nerve/chiasm abutment on MRI (or new symptoms to suggest this)
- Biochemical analysis in macroadenomas at 6 months and yearly after this (no need to recheck in microadenoma in the absence of clinical signs)

What Medical Treatments and When

Prolactinoma

- Best treated medically with dopamine agonists, dopamine agonist mandatory for tumor growth control in macroprolactinoma (i.e., >1 cm diameter), where in microprolactinomas dopamine agonist treatment is only indicated if clinical signs and symptoms are present (e.g., amenorrhea, hypogonadism) or if tumor continues to grow.
- Most commonly used are bromocriptine and cabergoline.
- Cabergoline is favored as it is more potent and has fewer side effects.
- 90 % success rate.
- Treatment needs to be lifelong in most patients with macroprolactinoma.
- Cessation of dopamine agonist treatment can be attempted in patients with microadenoma if no clinical signs and symptoms associated with hyperprolactinemia

are present, the tumor appears completely resolved on MRI, and serum prolactin is low normal for at least 2–3 years during continuous dopamine agonist treatment (recurrence of tumor and hyperprolactinemia in two thirds of cases).

• Primary surgical treatment should be avoided as always non-curative in the macroprolactinoma scenario, and potential damage of pituitary function can be avoided by dopamine agonist treatment in the microprolactinoma scenario; surgical intervention is only very rarely required if treatment resistance to dopamine agonists (including reserve drug quinagolide) occur or in the scenario of a macroprolactinoma with acutely compromised vision and no clinical response to dopamine agonists within 24 h of drug administration.

GH Excess (Acromegaly)

• Surgical treatment (generally chosen as first line).
• Somatostatin analogs can be used in case of disease not amenable to surgery and are also sometimes used for primary medical treatment of acromegaly; the drug causes a decrease in growth hormone production in 50–60 % of patients with a reduction in tumor size in up to 80 % of patients:

  – These medications can cause gastrointestinal side effects in 50 % of patients and gallstones in 20 %.
  – Sandostatin LAR (octreotide) 10–30 mg or Somatuline Autogel (lanreotide) 60–120 mg is given once monthly and costs about £10,000 a year.

• The growth hormone receptor antagonist pegvisomant is another option. The drug reduces IGF-1 levels in up to 90 % of patients (the GH level is not reduced):

  – Needs to be given by subcutaneous injection daily, expensive (up to £54,000 a year)
  – Most effective treatment for control of GH

• Dopamine agonists can be used but much less effective; only 15–20 % patients have reduction in GH (might be used if acromegaly and hyperprolactinemia concurrently present)
• Stereotactic radiotherapy/radiosurgery treatment (if primary surgery unsuccessful or disease recurrence and no amenable target for secondary surgery)

ACTH Excess (Cushing's Disease)

• Surgical treatment.
• Medical treatment aimed at inhibiting steroidogenesis can be used temporarily in preparation for surgery in particular in patients with severe glucocorticoid excess and related signs and symptoms (metyrapone inhibits CYP11B1 which catalyzes a key step in cortisol synthesis; ketoconazole, an antifungal that inhibits steroidogenesis;

in severe cases etomidate can be administered in non-hypnotic doses to achieve control of glucocorticoid excess, e.g., in Cushing-associated psychosis).
- Stereotactic radiotherapy/radiosurgery (if primary surgery unsuccessful or disease recurrence and no amenable target for secondary surgery).
- Bilateral adrenalectomy (if surgical treatment not successful, long-term medical treatment should be avoided as insufficient disease control in almost all cases and high risk of cardiovascular morbidity and thromboembolic complications in insufficiently treated Cushing's).

TSH Excess (TSH-Secreting Tumor)

- Surgical management mainstay.
- Can try somatostatin analogs.
- Beware drugs that reduce thyroid function (i.e., carbimazole) in the long term; can cause tumor growth.
- Beta-blockers may be needed for surgery due to hyperthyroidism.

Gonadotrophin-Secreting Tumor

- Surgical management
- No role for medical therapy

Role of Radiotherapy

Radiotherapy has a role in the treatment of pituitary adenomas and should be considered in the following circumstances:

- Inoperable disease (either due to extent of symptomatic tumor or health of patient).
- Failed medical or surgical treatment (i.e., functional adenoma not responding to medical treatment or tumor residuum/regrowth after operation).
- It can be particularly useful in acromegaly with failed medical and surgical treatment.

Depending on availability the options for radiotherapy are conventional radiotherapy (encompassing IMRT), stereotactic radiosurgery (i.e., gamma knife), or fractionated stereotactic radiotherapy (stereotactic radiosurgery as multiple doses). The side effects from all modalities are similar, with pituitary failure (up to 40 %), radiation optic neuropathy (up to 2.5 %), and secondary brain tumors (up to 2 %) occurring with each. At present stereotactic radiosurgery can only be used in small tumors away from the optic nerve/chiasm. Fractionated stereotactic surgery is a more novel approach with more research required.

Further Reading

Brada M, Ajithkumar TV, Minniti G. Radiosurgery for pituitary adenomas. Clin Endocrinol. 2004;61:531–43.

Freda PU, Beckers AM, Katznelson L, Molitch ME, Montori VM, Post KD, Vance ML, Endocrine Society. Pituitary incidentaloma: an Endocrine Society Clinical Practice Guideline. J Clin Endocrinol Metab. 2011;96(4):894–904.

Radiopaedia (http://radiopaedia.org/articles/inferior-petrosal-sinus-sampling).

The National Endocrine and Metabolic diseases information services (http://endocrine.niddk.nih.gov/pubs/acro/acro.aspx).

The Pituitary Foundation (http://www.pituitary.org.uk/content/view/208/).

Chapter 40
Hypophysectomy

Shahzada K. Ahmed, Rosalind Mitchell, and Alan Johnson

All pituitary surgery should be performed in specialist centers where all treatment options are available and where there is a multidisciplinary team approach.

The pituitary surgeon needs to counsel each patient with a careful explanation of the treatment options, with benefits and shortcomings of each, including the consequences of no treatment. Supporting literature is available from the Pituitary Foundation (www.pituitary.org.uk).

Indications for Surgery

- Mass effect
- Pituitary hormone excess not controlled by medical management
- Evidence of significant adenoma growth on serial imaging

S.K. Ahmed (✉) • A. Johnson
Department of Ear, Nose and Throat Surgery,
Queen Elizabeth Hospital Birmingham,
University Hospital Birmingham NHS Foundation Trust,
Mindelsohn Way, Birmingham B15 2WB, UK
e-mail: shahz.ahmed@nhs.net

R. Mitchell
Department of Neurosurgery,
Queen Elizabeth Hospital Birmingham,
University Hospital Birmingham NHS Foundation Trust,
Mindelsohn Way, Birmingham B15 2WB, UK

J.C. Watkinson, D.M. Scott-Coombes (eds.), *Tips and Tricks in Endocrine Surgery*,
DOI 10.1007/978-1-4471-2146-6_40, © Springer-Verlag London 2014

Mass Effect

Pituitary macroadenomas (tumors >1 cm in diameter) may cause visual loss due to direct pressure on the optic nerves and chiasm.

Pituitary Hormone Excess

Other than prolactinomas, which are treated medically, all other functional adenomas are effectively managed surgically. Rarely a prolactinoma that does not respond to medication may also need surgery.

Adenoma Growth

With the increased use of imaging, there are greater numbers of incidental pituitary adenomas. When these are small, do not cause mass effect, and are non-secretory, they are usually managed conservatively with surgery considered only if there is significant growth on serial imaging.

Local infection such as sinusitis needs to be eliminated before surgery to minimize the risk of meningitis.

Abnormal anatomy, such as a solid (poorly pneumatized) sphenoid, needs to be considered but is not a contraindication to surgery. Aberrant, ectatic carotid arteries can also occur. Intraoperative image guidance is invaluable in both these situations.

Surgical Approaches

The two main routes to the pituitary gland are transsphenoidal and transcranial. The endoscopic, transsphenoidal route is the method of choice in the vast majority of cases with a lower morbidity, although the transcranial approach is still indicated if there is a significant intracranial component inaccessible from below such as in some giant pituitary macroadenomas (Fig. 40.1). In such cases a staged operation with a transsphenoidal approach followed by a transcranial approach may be appropriate.

The sphenoid sinuses are variable in size and shape and are normally asymmetrical. Preoperative imaging gives the surgeon a map of the route to the gland. Image guidance can be very useful.

Endoscopic transsphenoidal route:

- The nasal cavity is decongested in the anesthetic room once the patient is anesthetized.
- The right middle turbinate is lateralized.
- The natural sphenoid ostium in the sphenoethmoidal recess is identified, and the anterior wall of the sphenoid on both sides is removed inferiorly and medially widening the ostium. The arterial branches supplying the nasal septum run

Fig. 40.1 Coronal T1 MRI showing a giant pituitary multicystic macroadenoma

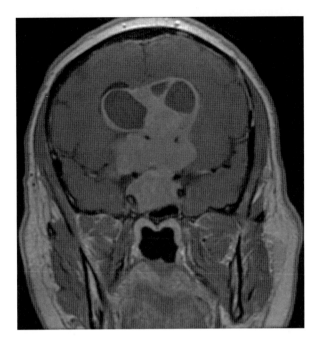

- inferior to the natural sphenoid ostium and are preserved by pushing the mucosa inferiorly, prior to bone removal, in case a future nasoseptal flap is needed.
- The posterior aspect of the septum is removed, approximately 1 cm anterior to the rostrum of the vomer, which is then also removed.
- A long shafted bur may be useful if the bone here is thick.
- Bone and mucosa are removed until a complete 360° view of anterior sella wall is achieved with at least an instrument width spare all around the pituitary fossa to allow space for instrument maneuverability during tumor removal (Fig. 40.2).
- The anterior bony wall of the pituitary fossa may be dehiscent, especially in macroadenomas, or occasionally (more commonly in microadenomas) be quite thick and needs drilling.
- The dura mater lining the pituitary fossa needs to be incised to enter the gland with sharp dissection, diathermy, or laser. A thinner layer of pituitary capsule is deep to this, and the surgeon may try to develop a plane between the normal gland and the tumor capsule. If there is brisk cavernous bleeding, it is likely that the surgeon has not completely cut through the dura. There are usually interconnecting venous lakes (superior and inferior intercavernous sinuses) that may need to be controlled with pressure, hemostatic agents, diathermy, or Ligaclips.
- If the tumor extends into the cavernous sinus, then it may still be possible to remove it in its entirety with wide exposure, angled curettes and a two-suction technique.
- In the event of a CSF leak, it is the authors' practice to seal it with a vascularized rescue nasoseptal flap harvested from the ipsilateral nasal septum. Most other techniques to repair CSF leaks in this scenario without using vascularized tissue have equally good results
- Complications

Fig. 40.2 Diagram of endoscopic view of the interior of the sphenoid sinus with the intersinus septum removed, showing the pituitary fossa (*PF*), optic nerves (*ON*), and internal carotid arteries (*ICA*)

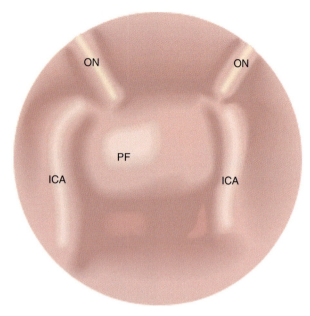

Intraoperative:

- Bleeding. The most common source of troublesome bleeding is the intercavernous connecting veins in the anterior capsule of the gland, which are easily controlled by packing. Hemorrhage from an internal carotid artery is a rare but potentially lethal complication if the artery is torn. This must be avoided by using only gentle blunt dissection or gentle suction and knowing where the arteries are from preoperative imaging.
- Cerebrospinal fluid leak. If a CSF leak arises during surgery, it is repaired at the time. If it persists or recurs postoperatively, it needs to be repaired before patient discharge, as described above.

Early postoperative:

- Diabetes insipidus (DI) is likely to occur when the pars posterior or pituitary stalk has been traumatized during surgery and may be transient in up to a third of patients but is persistent in up to 9 %. The diuresis normally begins on the first postoperative day, but a diuresis can occur for reasons other than DI, and so it is essential to monitor the serum electrolyte levels daily.
- Meningitis is rare but serious. Intraoperative antibiotic prophylaxis is always used as well as having a low index of suspicion.
- Significant intracranial hemorrhage is rare. If it is suspected from the clinical signs, it constitutes a neurosurgical emergency and should be managed accordingly.
- Pneumocephalus. Air may enter the CSF space if there is a CSF leak/skull base defect. If suspected, it can be seen on imaging (CT or MRI). Nurse the patient flat, and if it persists, repair any skull base defect.

Late postoperative:

- Anterior pituitary deficiency is detected on postoperative endocrine assessment and needs to be adequately treated with replacement hormone therapy.
- Pituitary surgery has a failure rate. In some cases, the abnormal levels of hormone will fall, but may not reach the criteria for cure. There is often a corresponding improvement in symptoms. The decisions on the need for and nature of further treatment are best made within the multidisciplinary team.
- Nasal and sinus complications are increasingly rare with endoscopic surgery, but sinusitis and nasal crusting can arise.
- Recurrence of the tumor can occur many years later. The standard postoperative protocol for these patients includes long-term follow-up.

Revision Surgery

The best chance of curing a pituitary adenoma is at the first operation. However, if cure is not achieved and the surgeon and endocrinologist feel that revision surgery is the best option, this should be done. If the first operation was a microadenectomy, removal of all or most of the remaining gland is likely to be appropriate unless the surgeon can easily identify an adenoma in the gland remnant, excise it and leave some normal anterior pituitary tissue. All series quote substantially lower cure rates and higher rates of hypopituitarism and increased complication rates in revision surgery. High-resolution (at least 3 T) MRI can often differentiate adenomas from normal gland and intraoperative image guidance is also extremely helpful.

Further Reading

Stell and Maran. Chapter 28, Pituitary tumours. 2012;528–42.
The Pituitary Foundation (www.pituitary.org.uk).

Index

Printed by Printforce, the Netherlands